You Can Feel
Better
Here's How

The guide for grown adults to lose weight, get stronger, bend and move better, and change that "old" feeling

By: Jeremy "tall trainer" Biernat

Disclaimer:

The information is book is meant to assist you not be your only resource. All exercises and health habits pose some inherent risks. (so does getting out of bed in the morning). Take responsibility for your own safety and health and know your limits. I'm not a doctor, nutritionist, or psychologist so please use those experts when you are considering this material. As for any exercise or dietary programs consult your doctor before using any of these strategies.

First Edition September 2024

For Bulk Purchases / Speaking Requests / Interviews please call us (585)260-4235

ISBN: 978-0-9980652-5-0

I want to dedicate this book to the millions of people who struggle with poor health and frustration with their bodies. I hope this helps.

Also, to my family, my co-workers in this mission, clients, and friends.

A biggest Thank you to God without whom I would not have enough passion, joy, or wisdom to rise out of my own selfishness.

- JB (the tall trainer)

Getting older?

Yep…me too…

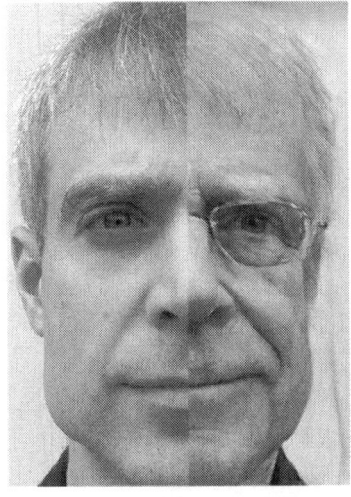

Of course, we are blessed for the chance to do so!

I want to get to the point quick so I'll keep this intro short. Afterall…we aren't getting any younger! But, what is younger?

I've been a personal trainer over 20 years now. My typical client is someone 50-70+ years old and I hear their struggles. What happens as we "age"?

- **We get fatter** – at a rate of merely 2 pounds per year it would make you 40 pounds heavier from 40 to 60 years old.
- **We get out of breath** – Things we used to do easy now make us sit down to catch our breath.
- **We get tight** – putting on socks has gotten harder to do. Getting into and out of things and up and down require heavy effort.
- **We get weaker** – we need to ask others for help with things we used to do ourselves.
- **We are in pain** – joints ache and the body hurts more places more often

I want you to know that these things can change. We can reverse most of the typical signs of aging. Maybe not 100% better but we can make significant improvements. I don't have a skin care routine so I'm not talking wrinkles. You can increase Strength, Stamina, Flexibility, Lose Weight, and generally feel awesome in less time than you think.

Most people think it will take monumental effort over years to see the benefits that are possible in months!

People are usually shocked when they see how much better they feel after only 4-weeks of our program. It's nothing crazy that we do. We just work to consistently apply the time-tested best practices for exercise and nutrition and amazing things happen!

For your benefit I'll be adding photos and stories throughout this book of some of our clients so you can be encouraged and perhaps a little more hopeful.

Basically, I want you to know that YOU CAN FEEL BETTER…

Now the rest of my time will be showing you HOW!

Real Results
"I am doing things I only dreamed of doing last fall!"

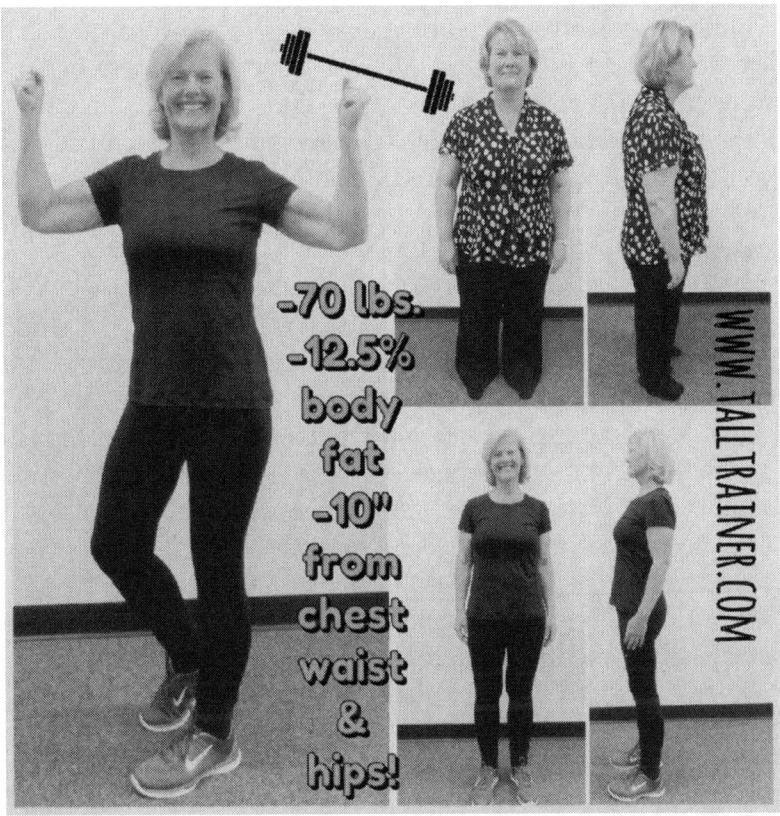

-70 lbs. -12.5% body fat -10" from chest waist & hips!

WWW.TALLTRAINER.COM

Last October I could hardly walk up a flight of stairs without becoming short of breath. I was tired and felt I was losing my edge at work. I tend to eat in response to stress. After back surgery, working full time while getting my masters in nursing, and being the primary caretaker for my mother with Alzheimer's I had gained a lot of weight –like 80 pounds!

As a Nurse practitioner I know too well the pain and suffering caused by inactivity and obesity. I see it every day. I knew how important exercise and weight loss were for my health, but

3

despite my best efforts I was not very successful at losing weight or exercising. Although it was hard for me to admit, I needed help.

In the past (many years ago) I was pretty good at showing up for exercise classes. I was trying to find an exercise class that would fit into my schedule when a newsletter from the Tall Trainer arrived in the mail. I wasn't sure the fitness classes were for me -boot camp sounded a little scary. I did a little more investigation on the Tall Trainer web site and learned that boot camp program seemed safe and doable, not extreme. It took me more than a few weeks, but I finally decided to make the call.

Best decision ever! What I found at Tall Trainer was a group of knowledgeable individuals who are truly committed to helping me achieve my goals. The nutrition advice and on-line nutrition program are excellent. You choose what you like to eat within healthy guidelines. I have lost 70 pounds in nine months and have not felt hungry or deprived. I am still surprised at how easy the weight loss has been.

When I first started I could not do all of the exercises, but was always given modified versions of the exercises that I could do. I never felt judged or out of place. The members are welcoming and supportive. Work outs are varied, fun, and effective. The structure and accountability of the program really works for me.

I am amazed how much improvement I have seen in my strength, endurance and aerobic capacity. I have more energy than I have had in many years. I sleep better. I feel sharper (the same exercises that are good for your heart are good for your brain). I walked up four flights of stairs at work the other day while carrying on a conversation – and did not think twice about it!

I am doing things I only dreamed of doing last fall. I completed a 5K race (ok, I mostly walked☺) and have signed up for a

4

paddle board course. It's really fun to see someone I have not seen in a while. I have changed so much that sometimes they don't recognize me. – Cindy

6

And so we begin…
How to Feel Better

I don't know how you feel about this but I feel like I want to live this life well. I feel like we are put on this earth on purpose for a purpose. I know for sure it's not to watch TV, or spend time double thinking life instead of living life, or to feel miserable the whole miserable time.

I've been around enough to see people who are in their 90's and active and helping others and loving every second of it. I've seen others in their 70's hoping to die soon to end the lonely, painful, misery they are in.

Similar to the shocking difference between these two:

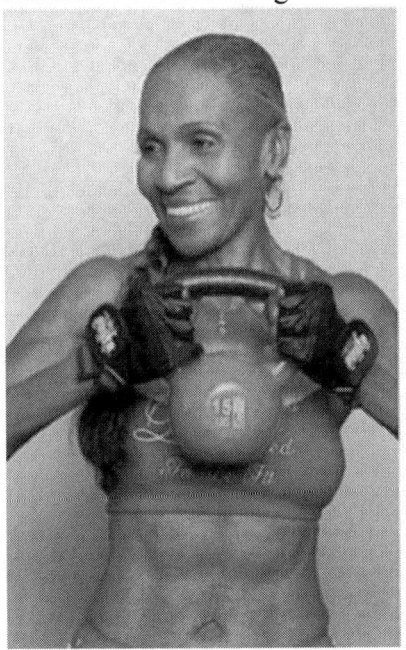 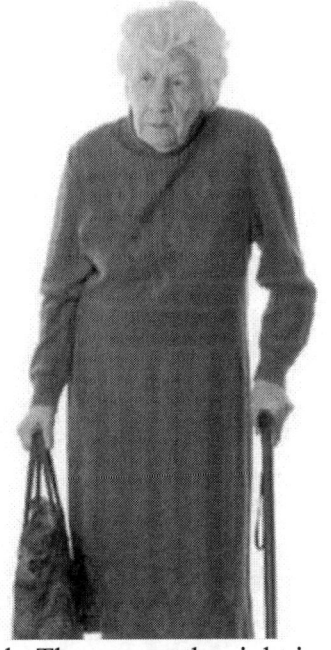

These women are both 80 years old. The one on the right isn't too bad off. In fact she is close to what we'd expect from 80 years old. The woman on the left (Ernestine Shepherd) makes

7

me question if I'm even in good enough shape for 80. She is physically leaner and stronger than a lot of 20-year-olds!

People like her inspire me to be different and see how well I can do this aging thing. I will promise you that she is following the principles I'm sharing in this book at a probably 90% or more consistency. If you don't need the abs I think you could be pretty happy doing these things 70-80% of the time.

Disclaimer: I'm an "exercise" guy and "nutrition" guy. I think they are amazingly powerful. But, They don't fix everything. The old quote says, "If all you have is a hammer everything looks like a nail." My main tools are exercise and nutrition and I apply them excessively and ruthlessly. But, they cannot stop all pain and hardships. What I have found though is that if terrible nutrition could make you feel worse then better nutrition could help you feel better. If no exercise can make your body sick and rot faster then adding exercise in could help you feel better. While exercise and nutrition cannot cure everything they can for the most part make a bad situation a little bit better. And sometimes all the way better.

So, if you are feeling in anyway like you could feel better and would like to feel better let's jump in to the first thing I think you should be doing.

Key #1 - Resistance Training

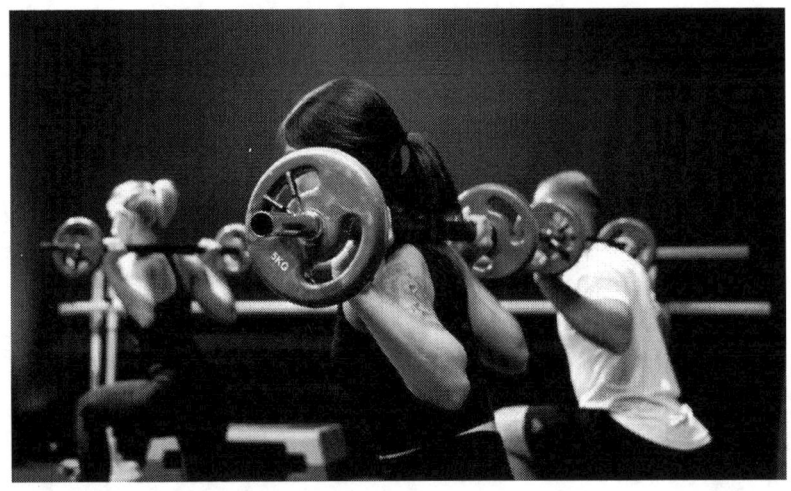

Resistance Training can help drop body fat, increase metabolism, improve flexibility, balance, strength, ability to do more activity in the day, also a mood booster!

There is amazing amounts of research on this now, but one of the most convincing to me was this one.

THE OLDER WE GET THE MORE IMPORTANT IT IS!

Resistance Training and Longevity
Melov, S. et al. (2007). Resistance exercise reverses aging in human skeletal muscle. PloS ONE, 2)5): e465.

In the study they took 26 people who were 68 years old on average and another group of 25 people who were 24 years old. They were all somewhat active and reasonably healthy before the study.

They did resistance training 2x/week for 26 weeks.

9

All the classic exercises.

Getting progressively heavier and more sets per workout.

They did muscle biopsies beginning and end. And did a mRNA analysis. Messenger RNA is a cousin of DNA. The DNA stays in the nucleus of the cell but the cell runs off of the information there. So the mRNA transcribe the DNA in the nucleus and then takes that message to the cell so it knows how to function.

The amazing results were…

179 GENES related to age and exercise had a reversal of gene expression (were functioning better!). **The gene expressions of the resistance trained older subjects was similar to the younger group in 179 different ways!**

It in a sense changed their DNA to younger!

The author of the study had this to say:

"We were very surprised by the results of the study… The fact that their **'genetic fingerprints'** so dramatically reversed course gives credence to the value of exercise, not only as a means of improving health, but **reversing the aging process itself**, which is an additional incentive to exercise as you get older." - Melov

So, for me this is a BIG reason to keep doing resistance training and if you aren't doing it currently it's hopefully a good reason to start!

68-year-old muscle more like 24-year-old muscle in 179 different ways!

This is not the only reason to build muscle.

The Mayo Clinic did a study in 2011 where 54 women were divided into 4 groups:

Group 1 – Diet w/weight loss
Group 2 – Exercise w/weight loss
Group 3 – Exercise without weight loss
Group 4 – Weight Stable control group

The women to exercised and did not lose weight still lost the same amount of **FAT** as the diet group who did lose weight!

The conclusion was – exercise without weight loss is still associated with a substantial reduction in total and abdominal obesity.

>>> This means the scale doesn't have to go down to get smaller. <<<

A real-life example…

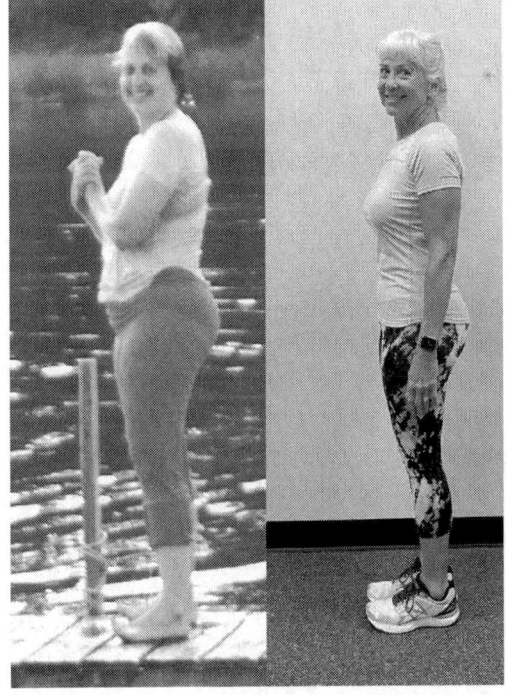

I remember my mom's weight loss story…actually she was one of the reasons I got into personal training. When I started as a trainer the profession was still considered something for famous people to pay for along with their private chef. **I saw my mom struggle through out my childhood with her weight and**

11

depression. 4 kids will do that to you.

The picture on the left almost cost my Dad his life. She almost killed him for taking it! She was not happy and nearly destroyed it, but she saved it as inspiration. She got down to her goal weight through a peer support group called TOPS – Take off Pounds Sensibly. A wonderful group for accountability. Well life happens. Her father, my grandfather, died and it kicked up a bunch of stress and tension in her family. She delt with the emotions through eating at times and gained some weight back. I started becoming her trainer and began working with her on resistance training. Which is one of the best reasons to get a trainer. **When she made it to the same weight again with resistance training instead of just diet only, she was SIZES smaller.** It was as if she had lost 10-15 more pounds. She was less fragile and better able to do many things.

Strength Training over Cardio

Many people are not sure how to do strength training so they don't.

They know they need to exercise so they go for a walk.

They would be infinitely better served using that time for strength training. There are just dozens more benefits. Most people walk for cardiovascular health or calorie burn. A 30-minute walk and a 30-minute strength training session would have similar heart rates and calorie burns. The only difference is afterwards the body has more work it does to recover (build stronger) from a resistance training session. It's like getting the benefit of the walk plus a whole lot more.

Don't get me wrong, a walk is better than nothing. It's just so much less beneficial than the same amount of strength training.

12

HOW TO DO STRENGTH TRAINING SAFELY

So, if we are sold on strength training here are my suggestions for how to go about doing it. We build these into our workouts in our training program.

One of the biggest fears people have is getting injured. It can happen and if you start exercising like I did by learning from friends or other people at the gym you might miss out on some critical learnings that can cause you pain, injury, and a loss of strength and conditioning while you recover.

The biggest thing I want you to know about strength training is posture. Most injuries in the gym are posture related. A lack of good posture while performing an exercise. To be clear I have seen dozens more people get injured in their regular life outside the gym than in. However, I have personally had aches, pains, and injuries because I did not value posture like I should.

If we use one of the most basic of exercises that most people know.

The Push-Up

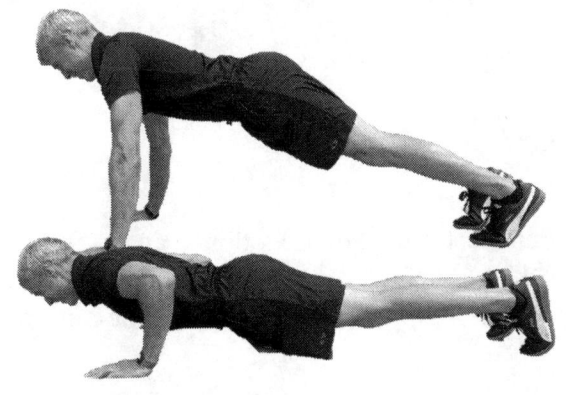

When we tell our bodies to get a job done it looks for the most efficient pathway. **If we have tight or weak muscles that pathway will undoubtedly run through the joint.** Putting extra pressure on our tendons, ligaments, cartilage, bursa sacks, and even bones. Some of these tissues can break or tear.

That's enough to make you want to skip the exercise all together. The only problem with that is we usually bring this bad posture into our unloading the car, yard work, or picking things up around the house. And we are more likely to have an injury in a deconditioned non-exercising body.

Our body is incredibly strong and incredibly fragile at the same time! We work very hard to create workouts to build on this strength while not increasing risks.

Most push-ups people scrunch their shoulders, flair their elbows out, pop their hips up, and/or drop their heads. Each of these positions puts more pressure on our rotator cuff muscles, tendons, and cartilage in the shoulder.

OUCH!

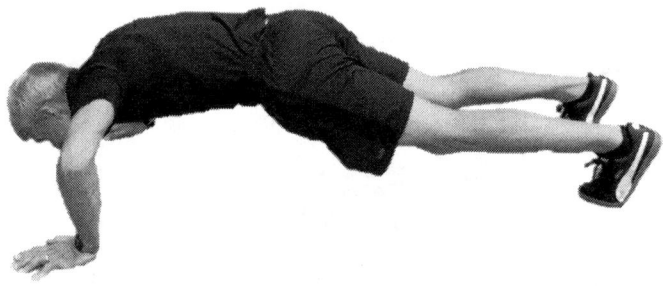

Getting the chest out, shoulders down (away from ears), chin pulled back, and armpit muscles flexing makes it an amazing exercise for strength, metabolism, and posture improvements.

NICE!

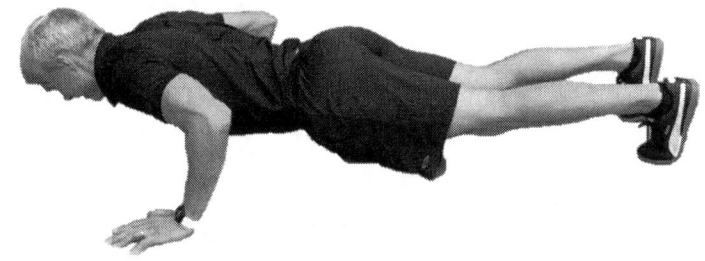

Our strength training exercises should be some of our best stretches. In good position and full pain free range of motion our bodies get looser than stretching alone can do!

So, strength training can improve posture, flexibility, burns at least as many calories as a brisk walk, Boosts metabolism for hours, improves our strength of course, and releases highly beneficial hormones into our body. To simplify...We feel soo much younger and better. It's worth it to learn how to do it right.

Each exercise has different pressure on the body and has different and common errors in technique. This is why I struggle to workout in a gym when other people are working out because I see the mistakes and even on vacation I feel like I should say something. It's common enough that if I walk into a full gym I could spot 5-10 errors before I can set my water bottle down.

This is why personal trainers have a job. It's simple enough to learn how to do it right but you have to take the time to learn it. If you aren't going to work with a trainer to learn these things you can simplify it by always trying to have great posture while exercising. The best I can do in a resource is the "BASICS OF EXERCISE" video available on www.talltrainer.com/the-basics-of-exercise

15

Basics of Exercise

hould be allowed to workout before they watch this resource!

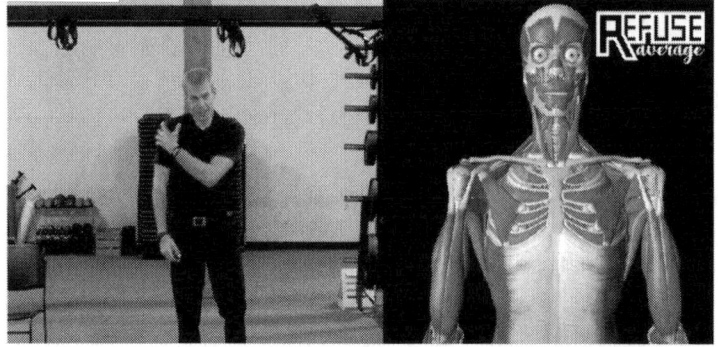

www.talltrainer.com/the-basics-of-exercise

**Scan with phone Camera
To go to website:**

If you watch this <30 min instructional video you'll know more about exercise than the majority of personal trainers! And I will feel better about you following ANY of my other advice or workouts!

Practical Guide to Strength Training
Muscle Groups / Movements

Generally you want a balanced and healthy body, right? To get this you'll want to work most of your muscles on a regular basis. Instead of talking about specific muscles I'll start with general movements.

Push
Pull

16

Squat

Are some of the most basic movements you'd want to be good and strong at. It's useful to train these using a variety of exercises so your body is more prepared for the less structured activities of life.

Volume, Speed, how much resistance, how many times, how many sets, how many days/week,

It can get super complicated which again stops people from beginning. There are arguments about all these things. When I started there were rules for this stuff that I didn't think made sense. I wasn't sure if they were true. Even in textbooks. Over the years I have been over joyed to find the rules I found to not be true have now been proven not fully true in research. Sometimes research informs practitioners and sometimes what we learn in practice get's studied and confirmed in research.

So, the biggest factors you need to actually pay attention to:

Working until your muscle stops being able to work or is close to this type of failure.
Do 10-20 sets per week per muscle group...for optimal results. Even 1 set per week can make changes if you have not been doing this type of work.

We've literally made hundreds of different workouts using these principles.

If I continue on just the push-up example here are some other versions of the same pushing action:

- Bench Press
- Dumbbell Stability Ball Press
- Band or Cable Press

There are ways you can even change up the basic push-up.

- Pausing at different places
- Moving Slower or Faster
- Changing your base – wide or narrow
- Using a suspension trainer, sliders, or stability ball
- And more…

These changes allow for your body to continue to strengthen the pushing action while giving the body some variations to help it be more balanced. And also you can keep working out without doing the exact same 6 exercises for the rest of your life. A little more fun too!

Every exercise has a correct posture, common errors, and ways to change it to keep it interesting.

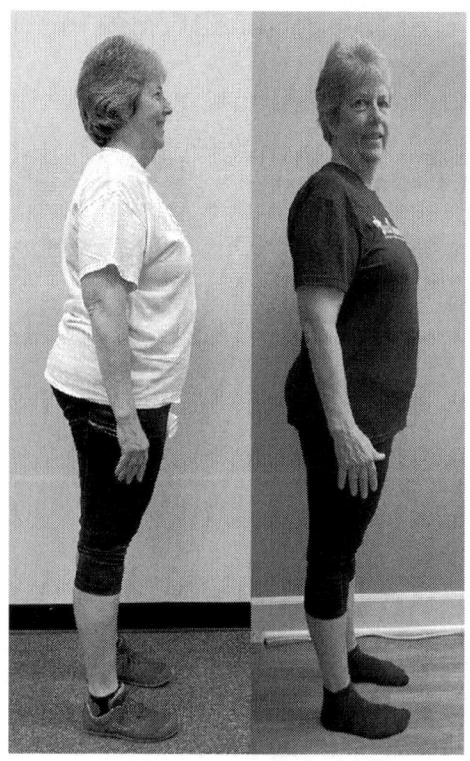

Sometimes you will choose an exercise because it is easier to do without hurting a damaged part of the body.

An example would be Terri. She has been wonderfully effective at weight loss and building strength even though she has a knee that is worn enough to be bone on bone instead of cartilage making things smoother.

The knee is not solved. It will probably need a

18

replacement to get "better". But, we used different exercises to allow her to access all the other benefits of exercise.

She dropped about 30 pounds in 3 months. Lost 5.7% Body Fat. And 6.8" at her waist!!!

Certain exercises are just not a good fit compared to others.

We work with people to find the best benefiting exercise without the potential negative side effects.

Some Helpful General Tips

2 rows for each press

Since slouching posture is so common it is considered good practice to favor the row or pulling action more than the press or pushing action. The idea is to do 2-3x as many pulling exercises as pressing to help rebalance the body.

Multi-Joint Exercises Before Single Joint

We don't hit this one all the time but generally it is good to do Multi-Joint Exercises like push-up (shoulder and elbow) before doing Triceps (elbow only). Many times we try to include some shoulder work even in the single joint exercise. It's just good practice to work on the harder to control exercises while you are fresh and have your best energy. Squats is considered a great exercise to start with as it is super challenging and fires up the body.

I think I'll leave this topic like this for now. You have enough info to get started especially if you watch the basics of exercise video. If you want to learn more you can join our group program or get help developing a strength training routine with some 1 on 1 training sessions. Usually takes 3 sessions to

19

develop a customized routine using the body you have and the equipment you have available. We do have an online program that has follow along workout videos but if you are local I'd feel better if you did a month of our program to learn how to do everything safely before jumping into that.

"The thought of having to take medicine..."

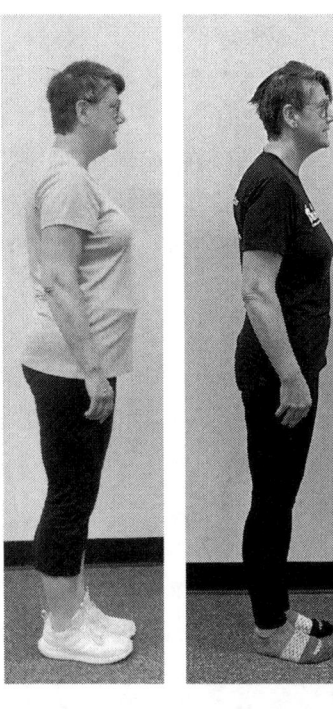
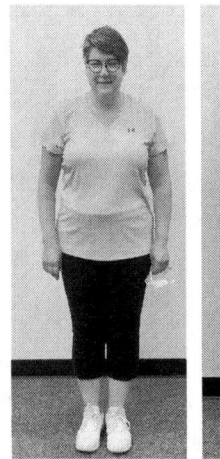
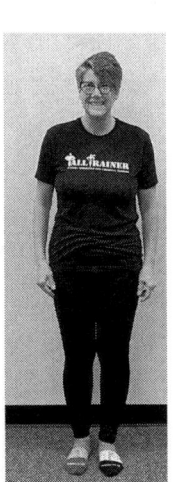

WWW.TALLTRAINER.COM

**-40 POUNDS
-6.2% BODY FAT
-8" @ WAIST
-5.5@HIPS!!!**

In December of 2021 I was diagnosed with high blood pressure. **The thought of having to take medicine for something I could help control did not sit well with me.**

So,I emailed Sarah and in January I set up some personal training sessions with Amanda twice a week.

21

In June of 2022, I started attending the daily 5:00 am class. (Amanda assured me I was ready and could do it!) **It was truly one of the best decisions ever. I absolutely love coming to class** (and truly like the people in my class) and enjoy whatever it may be that Jeremy has planned for us on any given day.

I have lost almost **40 lbs and feel so much stronger and so much more confident!** I love going to my closet and not having to try on outfit after outfit to find something that looks "good" or something to "hide" in. I love that when I went to the Luke Combs concert at Highmark Stadium and realized I bought tickets in the 37th row (nosebleed section!) that I didn't have to worry about climbing all those steps!

I am ashamed to admit that I didn't continue with Tall Trainer after my first free month because I thought it was "too expensive". *Nope! I'm worth it.* I also believe that if I weren't with Jeremy at Tall Trainer, I'd be doling out money for co-pays, doctor appointments, and various medicines.

My advice to anyone would be to take that first step and get started (you'll LOVE it), know your "WHY", and use your setbacks as opportunities for growth.

- Stacie

"In my younger years, I was physically active working at our family dairy farm. Then moved on to become a mechanic at Monroe Tractor for ten years. I had started getting issues with pain in my knees. I switched jobs to a position that was less physically demanding. As time went on, **my knees seemed to get worse,** as my weight fluctuated and **my diabetes was getting out of control**.

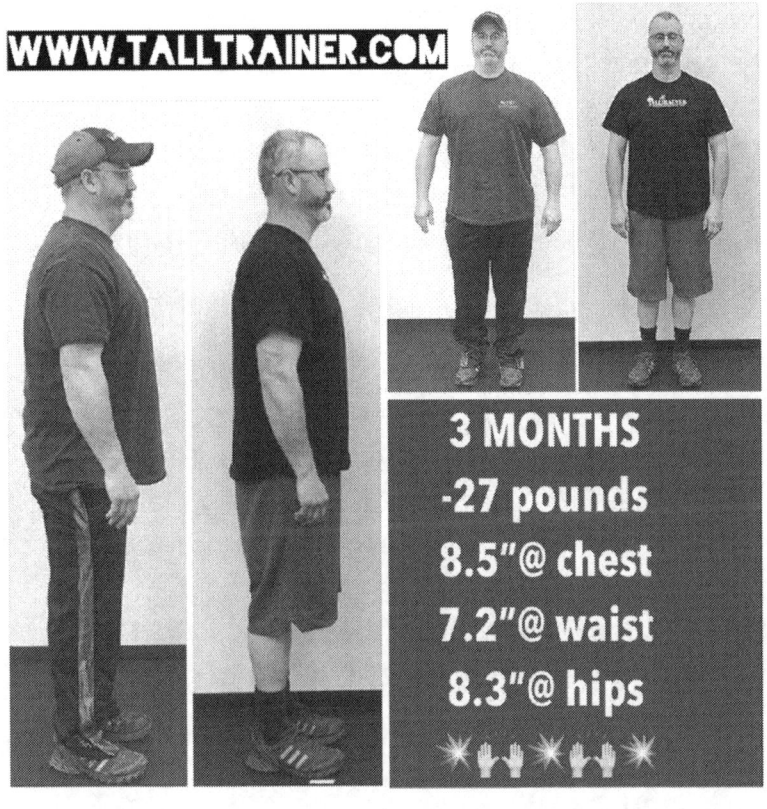

WWW.TALLTRAINER.COM

3 MONTHS
-27 pounds
8.5"@ chest
7.2"@ waist
8.3"@ hips

The thing that pushed me was when my wife got an opportunity to go to a boot camp style workout with some friends. I knew I wanted to do something to help

23

myself. I would like to say that **I am not the type of person that will just join a gym so this was a big step just walking through the door**. *I felt pretty down on myself, embarrassed of how weak and out of shape I had gotten.* Honestly, **I was actually afraid I could not make through the warm up the first day**.

The people at Tall Trainer really make you feel welcome and that you belong. Also the variety of exercises, equipment and Vitabot Food Journal make the whole experience successful. If you show up every day, do your best, and log your food, you will be successful! Jeremy shows you how to do each <u>exercise safely</u> so you do not hurt yourself. This was what I needed to get motivated and moving in the right direction.

When I started working out I was taking 1000 Mg of Metphormin a day plus another pill to help control my diabetes. I was also taking blood pressure medication . As of today I am down to 250Mg for my diabetes 1x a day . Hopefully in 3 months to be **completely off of medication**. I am more confident and have a lot of energy. **There are things I love to do now such as hiking and kayaking**. I have even been doing some jogging which is something I would never have done."

-   John

Key #2 – Resistance Training (and Body Fat)

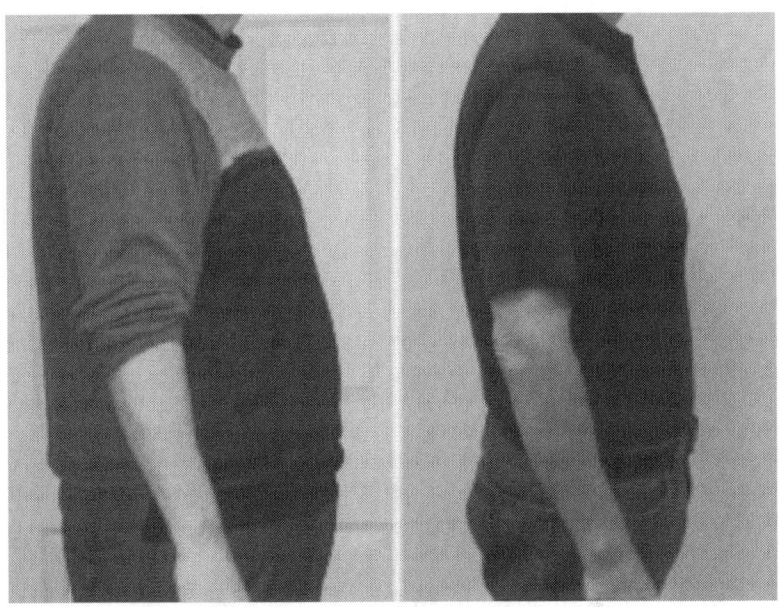

I know I already said resistance training is Key #1 but we are going to look at it a little more because I'm not convinced you are convinced yet. Even if you are ok personally with any extra weight you may carry. I will encourage you if you are heavier than necessary to lose even 10 pounds and see how this effects your blood pressure, cholesterol levels, endurance, strength, energy, body aches and joint pain.

To lose weight inspite of all the debate you still need to burn more calories than you eat. To lose 1 pound a week you need to eat 500 fewer Calories per day than what you burned in activity that day. For 2 pounds per week its 1000 Calories less.

25

This brings us to needed to talk about metabolism. Hopefully, I can demystify this a little.

6 Factors of Metabolism

There are 6 main factors that make up metabolism and really only 2 I want you to pay the most attention to. Metabolism is the rate at which our bodies burn through Calories.

1 – Age
2 – Gender
3 – Height
4 – Weight
5 – Activity Level
6 - % body Fat

The first couple aren't very encouraging to someone who feels their metabolism is slow.

1 – Age - simply increases only and with it some decline in metabolism. In a 59-year-old woman aging 20 years will make a 113 Calorie/Day drop in metabolism.

2 - Gender – a same height, weight, and all other stats man may burn about 114 More Calories than a woman. Not fair but that's how the stats go.

3 – Height - the shorter you are the lower your metabolism. This same woman increasing height from 5'5" to 6'0" would create a 38 Calorie increase in daily Calories burned

So the first three variables you have no control over. You were genetically gifted and chronologically gifted these. So they do factor in but not as big as the two factors I want you to work on.

4 - Weight - you do have some ability to change this variable. Unfortunately it works the opposite way than you wish. A 200

pound person would burn 263 MORE calories than a 150 pound person. Sometimes we feel the skinnier person must have a higher metabolism. Not true if both people have the same values in the other measurements. This means as you lose weight you burn fewer Calories doing the same things.

Ok, now the two I want you to pay attention to most:

5 - Activity Level - is the biggest factor by far. If you remember the Big Weight Loss Tv Show activity level is how they got most of their ridiculous results. If a 5'5" woman goes from Sedentary to Moderately Active (like doing an additional 10,000 steps/day). They would burn 465 more Calories! If they went to Extremely active (additional 25,000 steps) they would burn an extra 930 Calories! That is very hard to do but some people find this easier than cutting back too far on eating.

6 - % Body Fat is the final factor. If we carry more muscle on our bodies we will have a higher metabolism. This increases even more if we put that muscle to hard work regularly. I think this factor is one of my secrets to maintaining my weight so consistently. So a 12% drop in body fat at the same body weight would mean an increase of 228 Calories burned per day. Not as amazing as activity level but certainly worth some attention I would think.

Let's take a look at an example from research to see how we may have damaged our metabolisms.

Why Yo-Yo Dieting Stinks
AKA
Have you noticed how it's easier to gain weight back than it is to lose it?
International Journal of Obesity and Related Metabolic Disorders
1997; July 21(7): 574-9

27

e on a VLCD (very low calorie diet)
.verage of 19 pounds in 8 weeks (2.38 lbs a week)
32% of it was lean muscle tissue!
For Every 13 lbs of Fat Lost,
6 lbs of Muscle was lost!

If we follow this example and apply it to a typical dieter we'd get some graphs like this:

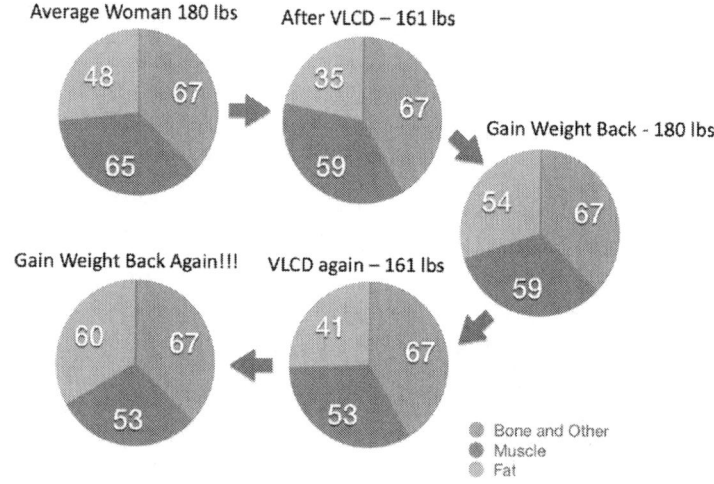

So this person drops the 19 pounds but falls off the diet and since they aren't doing any strength training they gain the weight back and they don't gain the muscle back. So now they have 6 more pounds of fat. If they repeat this another cycle they can now have 12 more pounds of fat AT THE SAME BODY WEIGHT!!!

28

To me this is shocking.

About 106 Calorie/day Drop in Metabolism because of lost muscle. Now eating the same foods this person can gain 10 additional pounds without any more indulgences.

This is why many people get frustrated with this process.

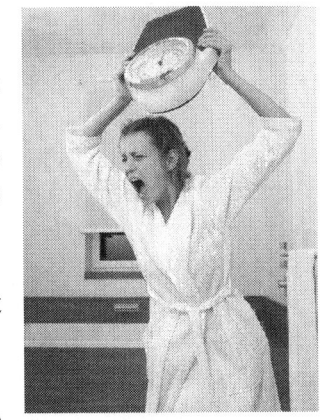

What if you want to lose weight but you do Strength/Resistance Training for your muscles while you do it? What happens then?

Answer = Good

Donnelly et al. Muscle hypertrophy with large-scale weight loss and resistance training. American Journal of Clinical Nutrition. 1993 Oct;58(4):561-5.

It used to be said that you can't gain muscle while losing weight because the body is in "break stuff down mode" not "build stuff up." Now if your top goal is muscle building I think you should look at % body fat and waist circumference more than the scale initially. If your top goal is weight loss but you still want muscle I think this study shows it can happen!

Participants were on a miserable 800 Calorie Liquid Diet for 90 days!! (not recommended and not fun, 3 months of not chewing?). I would say most people on restrictive plans this intense are usually back at their previous weight at the end of the year.

Average weight loss in the study was 35 lbs (2.92 lbs/week). Well above the recommended 1-2 pounds per week considered safe and more muscle sparing weight loss.

They did regular strength training sessions only. No cardio or they might have passed out!
"all subjects increased the cross sectional area of their muscle fibers significantly."

Conclusion = It appears that weight training can increase muscles (and therefore increases in metabolism) even during severe energy restriction and large scale weight loss.

More simply put...
Lift Weights = Increase in muscle no matter what!

So, don't take this as a recommendation. But, they should have lost tons of muscle like the other group but they didn't because of the resistance training. If you are losing weight. Do strength training. If you are gaining weight do strength training and some might be muscle! If you are maintaining weight do strength training!

Want to be an 80 or 90 year old who moves and feels like a 60 year old or better?

Just do strength training no matter what!

"I was nonexistent as a person - I was at the heaviest I've ever been in my entire life. **I had given up because I was so heavy."**

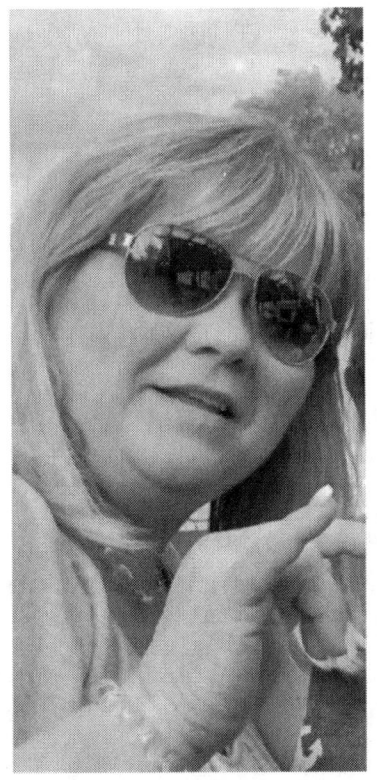
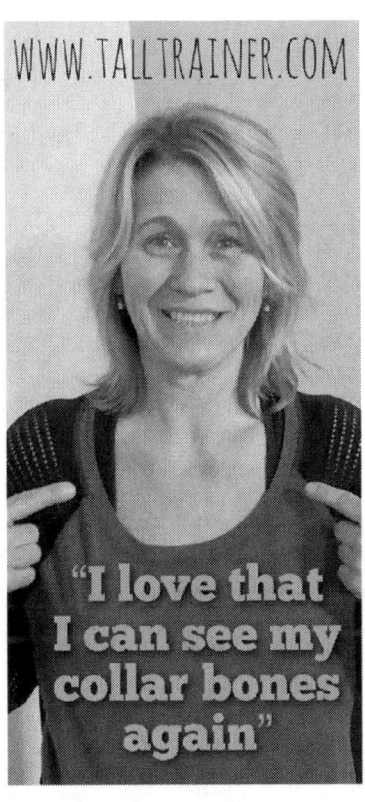

WWW.TALLTRAINER.COM

"I love that I can see my collar bones again"

"In June 2019 I decided to start, my son was getting married so that was my motivation join Tall Trainer.

At that point **I was nonexistent as a person** - I was at the heaviest I've ever been in my entire life. **I had given up because I was so heavy.** I felt like I was never going to be able to do it.

31

I was almost embarrassed to come in. In my head I thought everyone was in good shape there. I didn't want to be measured and have to be accountable.

But, I just got to a point where I was like *I have to do this! I have to put all of that aside*. The scariest day was the first day I started Tall Trainer. I hadn't stepped on a scale in I don't know how long. There was a lot of truths that day. I had to face what I actually weighed and that was a big "smack".

It was like *"wow, I let myself go there"*.

That was the LAST day I thought of it that way and decided to take off and have LOVED it!

In the beginning I had so much weight to lose I didn't struggle because the weight was falling off so quickly. I had a tool box that was given to me and set me up for success. The nutrition program, all the talks, and the personal phone videos sent to me on Fridays. Everything was always put into place for my success. It was me just putting in the work. It was easy in the beginning because the first four months I think I lost 16 pounds every month -so seeing and that was wonderful!

When it started slowing down I had to come to terms with readjusting as my weight loss changed. But along the way Jeremy was so good about showing me how to change according to my weight and what I needed to do with my nutrition. I always felt like I had a

<u>cheerleader</u> along the way and that was so important to me.

I have now lost **131** pounds and over 21 inches at my waist and hips. That has been so fun! <u>I also love that I can see my collar bones again!</u>

I can run up steps now. I work at an elementary school building and I go up lots of steps. I remember having to stop and wait a minute to catch my breath and now I just glide.

The feeling of "lightness" is my favorite part. I feel a bounce in my step, I don't get as tired, I want to go for walks and go do something. <u>My whole family has changed</u>. Even my son has lost 75 pounds.

If you're someone new wanting to start, **It's NEVER too late**. I'm in my 50s and I did this. I wish I didn't wait so long to do this. GIVE IT A TRY. It's definitely worth it. It doesn't always feel like exercise. This is fun. I get up at 5 every morning and do this and I am not a morning person. The rewards are defiantly worth the 5am wake up."

-    Kris B.

-

"Over the past 9 months I have lost 55 pounds and inches all over my body and an amazing amount of fat.

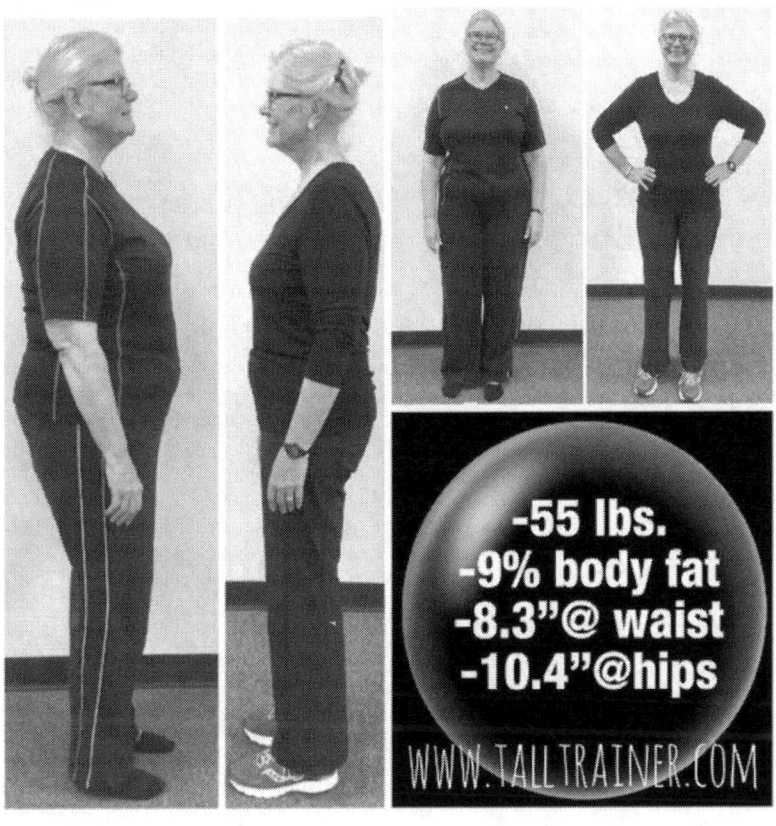

-55 lbs.
-9% body fat
-8.3"@ waist
-10.4"@hips

WWW.TALLTRAINER.COM

I've had to go through my closet twice to remove the oversized clothing – a great feeling! I've gained strength, balance and energy! I have more energy and have finished six 5K races (walking) this summer, I am more active than I have been in years and feel better too! I am looking forward to racing our sailboat next year, as I know I'll enjoy the experience so much more.

When I started Tall Trainer nine months ago, I had been fairly inactive for a long time; and my eating habits were none too healthy. I had been telling myself for quite a while that I needed to get back in shape, but I couldn't seem to get started. Now in my 60's, I realize that I want to be (and need to be) in good shape as I age and enter my seventies and beyond.

My inspiration for starting was just that I was tired of being tired and overweight and not able to do things the way I used to do and I wanted to do once again: walking, sailing, hiking, etc. A friend, who had been attending Tall Trainer, mentioned the group to me at a Friday night party. Somehow the timing was right for me. I signed up the next day and started Boot Camp that Monday.

The journey has been amazing so far and it continues to be. The trainers are fantastic and accommodate any physical limitations (like my knee) by modifying exercises. The exercise routines vary from day to day and never get boring. My classmates are an awesome bunch. Having worked with them and been encouraged by them for the past 9 months has been a tremendous boost to my motivation. Also, Vitabot, the nutrition-tracking program we utilize, is great. I use it every day as I plan meals; and I love the instant feedback on the choices I make – no guessing involved there.

One thing that I've learned and want to share with you: Don't wait for that "magic moment" - that

36

moment when the stars are aligned and you feel "This is it, I'm finally ready to start getting healthy and fit". That moment may never come. So, just do it - do it now - for you.

If you are thinking about joining the Tall Trainer Boot Camp, you should definitely try it. You will be amazed at what you can do, especially with all of the support you will receive from your trainers and classmates."

- Maggie

Key #3 – FOOD QUANTITY (ok also quality)

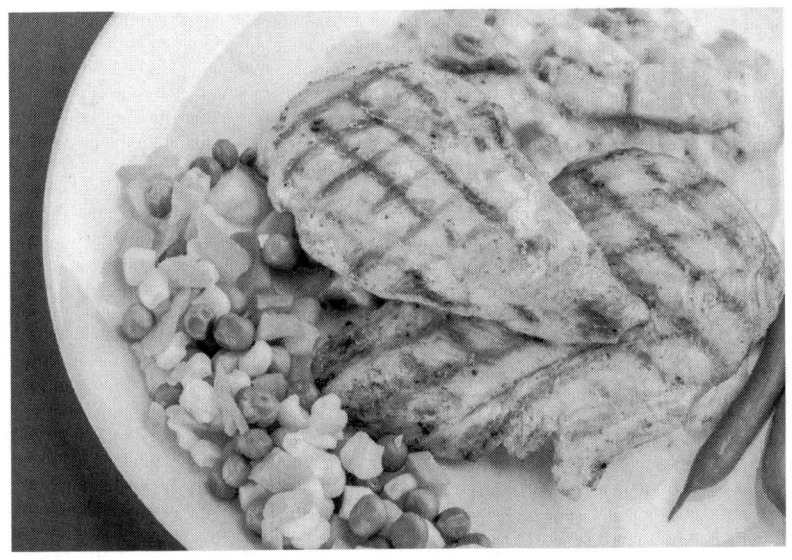

Let's jump into some more on nutrition. Dieting!

DIET

A 4 letter word!!!

In the classic sense diet is the typical food intake of a person or animal. We all have a diet and its either helping our bodies or hurting our bodies.

There is a lot of confusion in this area. Thousands of diet books. VERY conflicting often **OPPOSITE** recommendations!

Let look at the mess and then I'll attempt to clean it up and clarify it and give you some simple recommendations.

Let's look at a couple popular titles around currently:

Paleo
Vegan
&
Keto

I'm going to try to do this without BASHING any one of them. I just want to give you the full truth and leave you with the most basic steps I can.

First up Paleo

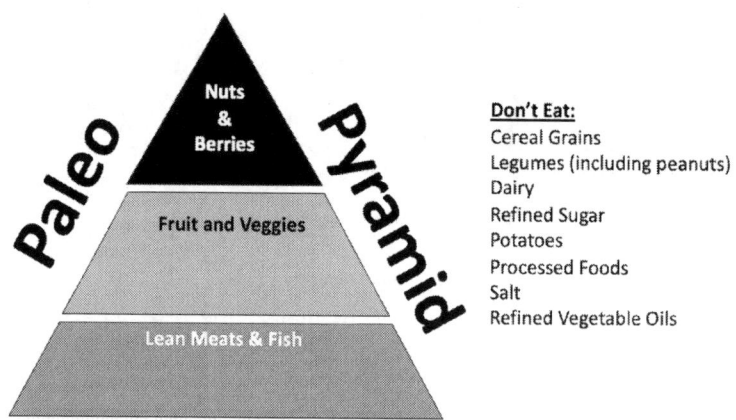

This diet is focused on eating like primitive people. Hunter/Gatherers. You can see they are eating mostly things that are found in nature and not things that take much if any processing.

For these examples I want you to notice the bottom of the pyramid for each. This is the eat a ton of this category.

Ok Without too much comment I'll jump to Vegan.

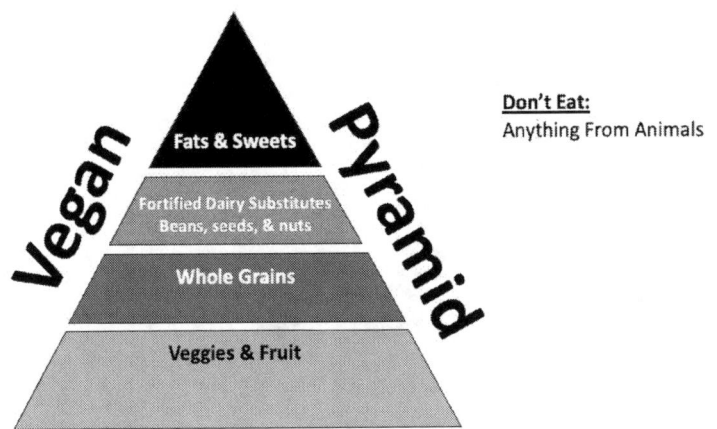

This diet is focused on eating plants only. In some ways easier to figure out since there isn't a list of foods just eat plants not animals. Most people that eat this way are dangerously low in protein and their muscles are not doing well because of it. It is possible to do this with adequate protein but requires more attention. Notice the bottom of the pyramid is the same as the second level on Paleo. But Vegan has Grains in second level and there are no grains in paleo diet.

Last but not least is Keto.

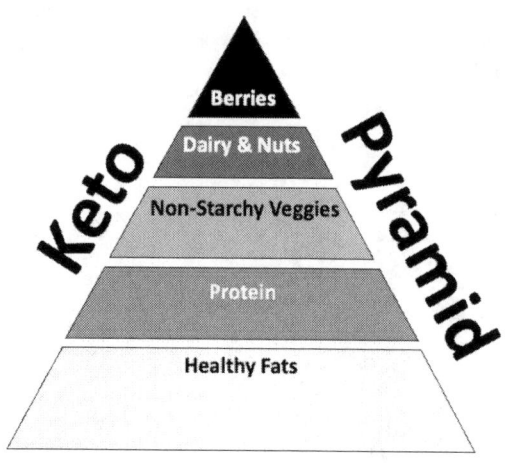

This one is Adkins revisited. It's about eating less carbs, which in general I'm in favor of. I'm just not sure you HAVE to cut them so far to get a benefit. Basically, that's the big point no carbs or sugars for the most part. Vegetables can be leafy, broccoli type, or green beans, etc, No wheat, corn, peas, potatoes, or even most squash. The base of the pyramid is FAT! Surprising to many who feel that fat is what's killing us. I think it's possible to do this in a mostly healthy way with some small tweaks. Zero Grains again and almost zero fruit which makes this one unique.

Three very different philosophies on nutrition. There are hundreds more but hopefully this comparison will help you as you observe other "new" trends.

The big disagreements in these 3 are:
- EATING MEAT
- EATING GRAINS
- EATING CARBS

I think disagreements are not where the real truth is found. People have lost weight and felt better on ALL 3 of these diets so let's instead look at the many agreements of the healthiest paleo, vegan, and keto.

42

At their best they all agree…

- Organic Vegetables are a large portion oɪ ᴄ.
- Avoid Processed Food
- Eat whole foods as close to nature as possible
- Nuts and some fruit is good

So when I look at all this what do I decide to do?

Me (Jeremy) says:
Eat a BUNCH of vegetables
Eat some meat because it's super hard to get protein without it
Eat light on grains, sugars, and nuts
Strangely enough don't go too crazy on fruit

You don't HAVE to follow my distilled recommendations. We've had many people do very well in our program NOT eating any vegetables. Not eating Meat. Etc.

But, here's the 6 BIG Nutrition Targets that you should try to hit no matter what "DIET" regiment you are following.

6 BIG Nutrition Targets

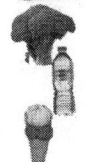

1. Protein
2. Eat every 3-4 hours
3. Eat <u>some</u> Fat still
4. 2 pounds of veggies
5. ½ of your body weight in OZ of water.
6. One HIGH Carb day per week

This is the pretty picture version of the list. Each of these points has proven itself VERY POWERFUL over my 20+ year career

43

way smarter people than me have spent their careers on just e of these 6 points. If you could do these 80% of the time you'd make steady progress. 90% and it would be FAST progress.

I'll break this down a little bit for you while still keeping it short. This could be a book on it's own.

#1 – Protein - .64 to .9 grams of protein per pound of body weight. Example: 150 pound person would be shooting for 96g – 135g of protein per day) 83.2– 117

This puts you at needing to take in at least 20 if not 30 grams per meal.

Now this is 30 grams of Protein not 30 grams of chicken. 100 grams of chicken breast (3.5 oz) has about 31 grams of protein in it.

This recommendation level is for muscle building. If you didn't have a goal to build muscle you could do less than this. It turns out as we age muscle actively tries to leave our bodies making us more frail. Without a high enough protein level your chances of gaining muscle back are slim.

This point is probably the most important nutrition target for success in shaping your body and losing weight. It turns out this level of protein is super filling too allowing you fewer cravings throughout the day. If you are convinced you need to do strength training from earlier you'll need to get the protein in to get the full benefits of the work you are doing.

If you aren't sure how to get started on this we made a couple resources for that too.

44

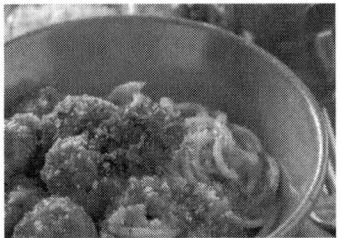

Hopefully these will give you some ideas for getting started. In our program we work more individually with you to help get a nutrition program going that works best for your unique situations.

#2 – Eat every 3-4 hours and more at the start of the day

This point is big for controlling hunger. You need to eat before you get TOO hungry. If you get too hungry the healthy food sounds worse to eat and the only thing you'll really want is carbohydrates (sugars or breads). Eating a bigger breakfast consisting of about 30 grams of protein will start you off in a much better hunger situation. Some people will say…but I'm not that hungry.

id! Eat before you are! What if we could stay not that hungry more of the day?

There are a couple factors at play here. They are so used to the ravenous hunger that they wait too long until they feel that hollow hunger, while thinking they are helping their weight loss chances. Also, it could be true that they eat too much at night and they do have some carry over from that.

Either way it's still good to get that protein started at least.

If you miss your protein level in breakfast that would mean you might need 50 grams for lunch and 50 grams for dinner. Which is harder to eat in one sitting.

Also, the "good" foods take longer to digest so you need to eat them before you get "super hungry", otherwise you will still be hungry after your meal and be tempted to over indulge.

#3 – Eat Some Fat Still (about 10 grams per meal)

Fat is filling. Fat also has TONS of calories. I know many people who have failed at their nutrition and weight loss goals because they ate too many almonds. Also, all our favorite indulgences for the most part have a high fat level. It can be hard to lower this. However, most people when they switch into "DIET" mode cut out too much fat.

Most of our clients need about 30-50 grams of fat for the day. If you spread it out so you are more satisfied throughout the day you'll be taking in about 10 grams per meal.

When you have that 10 grams ish per meal the food is more filling and you can absorb the fat-soluble vitamins A, D, E, and K. Too much below this mark and you won't get those two benefits. Too much above this mark and you'll struggle to keep your calories in a weight loss or non-weight gain level.

46

If you get this one wrong you'll notice it in the meal after where you are significantly more hungry. Which will tempt you towards the Carbs.

#4 – 1 pound of raw and 1 pound of cooked veggies

I realize this is an absurd number for most people. Many people the largest vegetable serving they have is the lettuce and tomato on their hamburger. I'm sharing with you ideal targets. Sometimes these get watered down so people feel better about trying to hit the strive for 5 etc.

The bottom line on this one is we were designed to eat mostly vegetables and some meat. Not pasta, chips, pizza, cookies, and ice cream. I still eat all the "bad" foods I just listed but not as often and not as much.

I think we'll be much better off focusing on what we **ARE** going to eat instead of what we are **NOT** going to eat. I saw this recommendation first from Dr. Joel Fuhrman author of "Eat to Live". The pound of cooked is recommended because raw vegetables are a big job to digest. You do have to do a lot of chewing to break them down.

Some people will say, "Vegetables hurt my stomach". I find it's often that they also forgot to chew them. They tried to swallow them after 3 chews like a fast food burger. An entire piece of broccoli is not supposed to make it into your stomach! That might cause some in-digestion!

I've tested this 2 pound of vegetable recommendation by using our food journaling software. I figured if this is a good recommendation then if I have 2 pounds of vegetable I should be able to have a bunch of junk for the rest of the calories and my nutrition scores should be good. So I added a pound of broccoli and a pound of romaine into the program. Then

47

because it's one of the most well known foods I decided to add pizza. I thought "wouldn't it be funny if you could have a whole pound of pizza?"

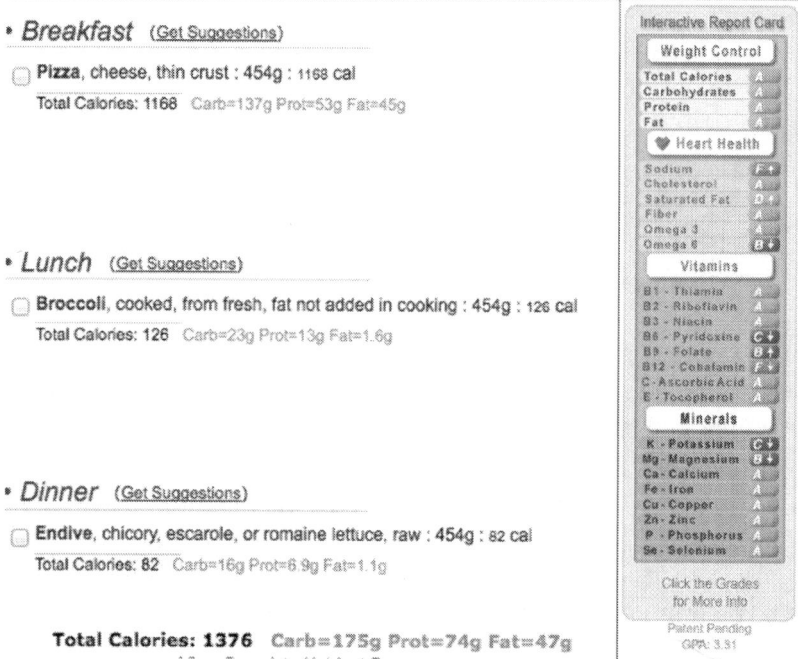

• *Breakfast* (Get Suggestions)

☐ **Pizza**, cheese, thin crust : 454g : 1168 cal
    Total Calories: 1168 Carb=137g Prot=53g Fat=45g

• *Lunch* (Get Suggestions)

☐ **Broccoli**, cooked, from fresh, fat not added in cooking : 454g : 126 cal
    Total Calories: 126 Carb=23g Prot=13g Fat=1.6g

• *Dinner* (Get Suggestions)

☐ **Endive**, chicory, escarole, or romaine lettuce, raw : 454g : 82 cal
    Total Calories: 82 Carb=16g Prot=6.9g Fat=1.1g

Total Calories: 1376 Carb=175g Prot=74g Fat=47g

It actually worked!! Here it is. 1376 total Calories. Protein is a little low at 74 grams but not bad. You can see the grades in the column. Lots of A's. Better grades than most health freaks can get with their fancy expensive foods.

This was such an Aha moment for me.

You don't have to be perfect...You just have to get enough good stuff in!

I mean there is only 208 Calories from Vegetables! 1,168 Calories of Pizza! But the mass of vegetables came through.

If you are interested in longevity (like being an amazing 80 and 90 year old), or you want to hedge your bets on Cancer (lots of studies on veggies), Feel full and satisfied for most of the day,

48

and flood your body with energy and vitality. You might want to look into these vegetable things!

#5 – ½ of your body weight in Oz of water. 150-pound person would drink 75 oz of water.
We all know water is an essential fluid. Most of us don't drink enough and simultaneously think we drink more than we do! I like this recommendation because it factors in body size. Vs the 8 x 8 oz glasses of water (64 oz).

Water helps our bodies to function better. As dramatic as cholesterol improvements and decreasing pain. It takes up physical space in the stomach which can help you be more full too. Our hydration and hunger signals can get confused. We get a strange stomach feeling that can be confused with hunger and cause us to eat more.

Many good reasons to try to get this quantity of water. Drinking slowly with occasional sea salt is probably best but sometimes you might need to chug it to make it happen.

#6 – One HIGH Carb day per week (+500-1000 Calories also)

This is one of the stranger recommendations from a personal trainer. Our normal eating should be lower in Carbohydrates. Especially when trying to lose weight or if we are not extremely active. The more active we are the more carbs we can have.

So, if we do low carbohydrate long enough our body starts to compensate. It lowers Leptin levels causing weight loss to slow. Leptin is the hormone that tells our body we have plenty of fat its ok to lose some. The only way to boost it is to actually get more fat OR eat one day like if you ate that way all the time it would be a problem.

The couple days after the high day are your peak fat burning days. Unfortunately this doesn't work when you do multiple

49

high days in a row like Friday, Saturday, and Sunday. It seems to work best with higher sugar type foods but it's a good time to eat a little of what you've been craving.

This effect is strongest the lower your body fat is. So the closer you get to your goal weight the more you'll need this target in place.

Food Quantity is more important than quality

When it comes to weight loss and arguably general health how much food you eat is more important that what foods you eat. I have had many clients who eat WAY healthier than I do but they are struggling to lose weight.

Let me show you a couple examples...

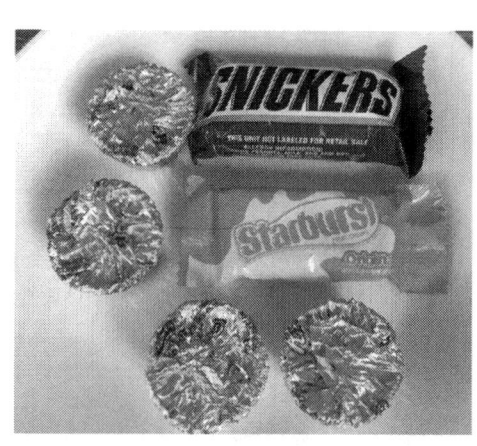

What if I told you...

You can eat all these candies...

Have 92 grams of Protein
Only 1368 Calories
AND a 4.0 GPA???

But wait there's more!

It sounds like a trick but they key is that this is not the only food eaten. There is enough good food happening and all the amounts are balanced. You could eat these candies every day and lose weight and improve health.

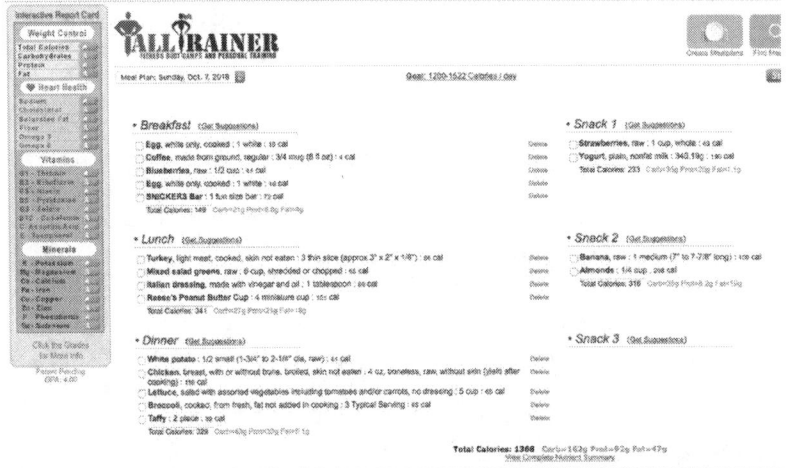

This is a screen shot from our nutrition program with these candies added with other foods. Snickers bar in breakfast. Lunch has the 4 peanut butter cups and turkey and 6 CUPS OF SALAD! That's a lot of salad. They are getting the 2 pounds in today! Dinner has the starburst (taffy), 5 Cups of Lettuce, 3 servings of broccoli, 4 oz of chicken, and even a small potato. This would be a harder meal to eat as there is no dressing on salad, no butter on broccoli, and nothing added to the chicken or potato. But, you got candy!

The reason this works is that because the candy is there you have to lower other foods. Lower them to balance out the candy.

Here's another example…

Twinkie diet helps nutrition professor lose 27 pounds

By **Madison Park**, CNN
November 8, 2010 8:40 a.m. EST

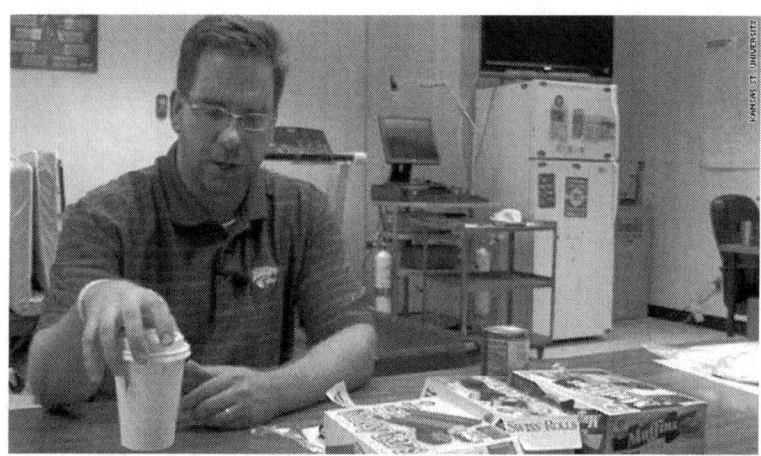

Mark Haub of Kansas State decided he'd use himself as a lesson to one of his nutrition classes. He had gained weight and needed to lose a little. He decided he wanted to show that quantity of food matters more than quality. So he planned to eat junk food. Vending machine food. Or many gas station food would be another way to mention it. He also wanted to eat this way because many people live in food deserts that make fresh fruits and vegetables almost impossible. He allowed himself a scoop of protein powder, a generic multivitamin, and a can of veggies along with his junk food.

In 2 Months he:
Lost 27 pounds
BMI 28.8, considered overweight, to 24.9, which is normal.
LDL, dropped 20%
HDL, increased by 20%
Triglycerides dropped 39%

How could this happen?

He knew exactly how many calories he was eating. And never went above that number! It was junk but it was a smaller amount than the healthier food he had been eating.

I cannot stress this point enough. Sometimes people think I will judge them by their food choices. Like I'll be mad if they eat a cookie. I actually don't care as long as the rest of the day is structured to fit in the calorie, protein, and nutrient ranges like the earlier candy example.

Not yet sure of this? Here's another example...

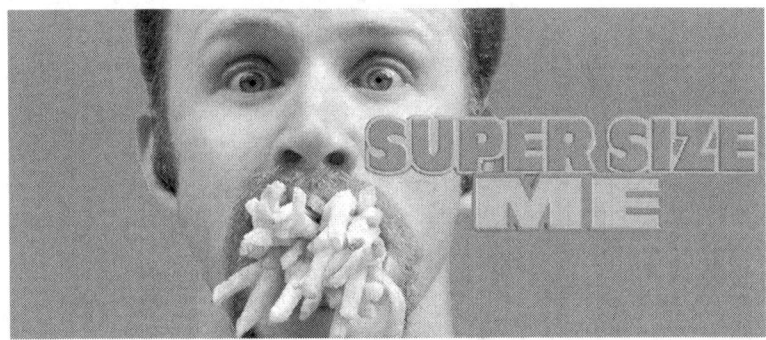

Most people heard about the Super Size Me Documentary. Morgan Spurlock challenged himself to eat McDonalds every day and super size the meal whenever asked. Just 30 days. He gained 24.5 pounds in 30 days! He also, required himself to only move just a few thousand steps per day to reflect the typical person.

This got us all thinking. Fast food is so terrible it's killing us all!

But most people didn't see this one!

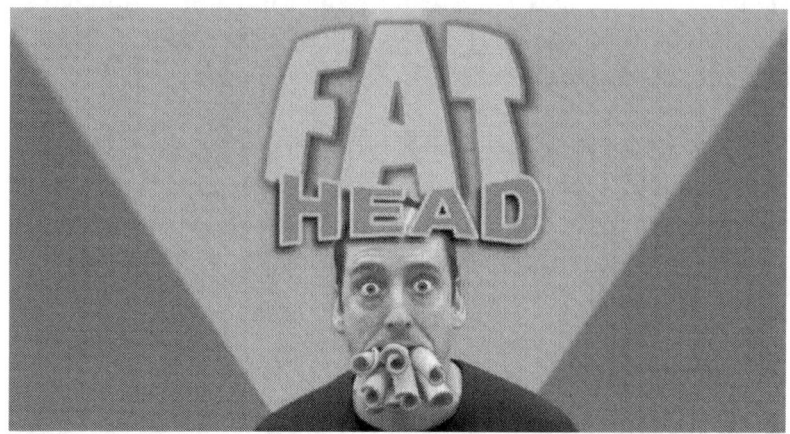

Tom Naughton thought the super size me documentary was over the top provocative. He contested that you can even lose weight on fast food. Because the key is how many calories are there! So he ate fast food every meal but planned out his menu to keep his calories in a weight loss range. He walked 6 days a week to get a little bit of activity. No dramatic workout routine.

He lost 12 pounds in the month and all his blood numbers improved also.

These examples along with my experience training people for the last 20+ years has cemented in my mind how powerful FOOD QUANTITY is vs FOOD QUALITY.

So, part of our program is a food journal. Just keeping track of what you eat. The key to this food journal is MEASUREMENT! How much is there!

A list of foods means almost nothing to me.

Oatmeal and berries for breakfast
Yogurt for a snack
Turkey sandwich and carrots for lunch
Big Salad with chicken for dinner

This list doesn't tell me the most important thing about food...HOW MUCH IS THERE!

Here's a shocking visual...

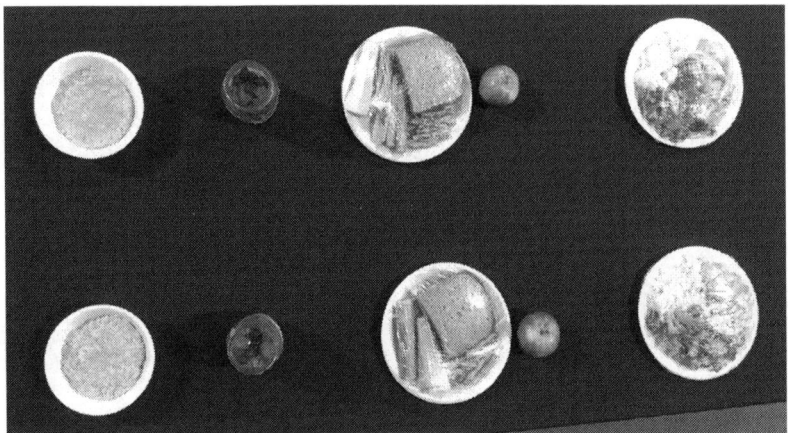

This picture has two example days. If you ate the top examples and your friend ate the bottom examples you'd both probably say, "we ate the same thing today."

BUT...

The top meals have only 1486 Calories
The bottom meals have 2358 Calories!!!

That's a 875 Calorie difference that is just attributed to how much food is there. There's just a little more of the high calorie ingredients in each meal adding up to a BIG difference.

I find people who think they are eating well can sometimes be 100 or even 200% wrong on their Calorie amounts!

They think they are eating 1200 Calories per day but they are actually at 2400!

Let's look at another study...

55

J Am Diet Assoc. 2002 Oct;102(10):1428-32.
Energy intake and energy expenditure: a controlled study comparing dietitians and non-dietitians.

Champagne CM1, Bray GA, Kurtz AA, Monteiro JB, Tucker E, Volaufova J, Delany JP.

They took 10 registered dieticians and 10 non-dieticians and had them keep a food journal where they even measured their food. Then they used Doubly Labeled water to get the actual calories and energy burn for the subjects. This is an expensive process which unfortunately keeps the sample size pretty small. But just imagine you were in this study. You knew they'd be able to tell EXACLTY how much you've eaten and burned. Wouldn't you be compelled to do your best 7-days of food journaling ever??? What if you were a dietician. I feel like your ego would not want you to be the worst dietician.

They worked hard yet look at what happened!...

The dieticians were off an average of 223 Calories per day. So if they thought they were eating 1200 calories they were actually eating 1423!

The non-dieticians did worse with an average of 429 Calories under-reported. So, the 1200 calories they thought they ate was actually 1629 Calories!

This amount of error is enough to think you are due a weight loss but get none at all.

I think this is super common except more extreme since we don't have the pressure of a short time window (7 days) and a study making us focus better.

If you aren't measuring your food you are most likely going to struggle with weight loss until you get serious enough to actually do it!

56

In fact if you want to lose weight but don't want to do a journal I'd rather you not join our program. Do something else for now. When you've had enough and are ready to do what it takes…including a food journal then please contact us! We are willing to work hard for you if you are willing to work hard too!

Here's a little bonus help along these lines…

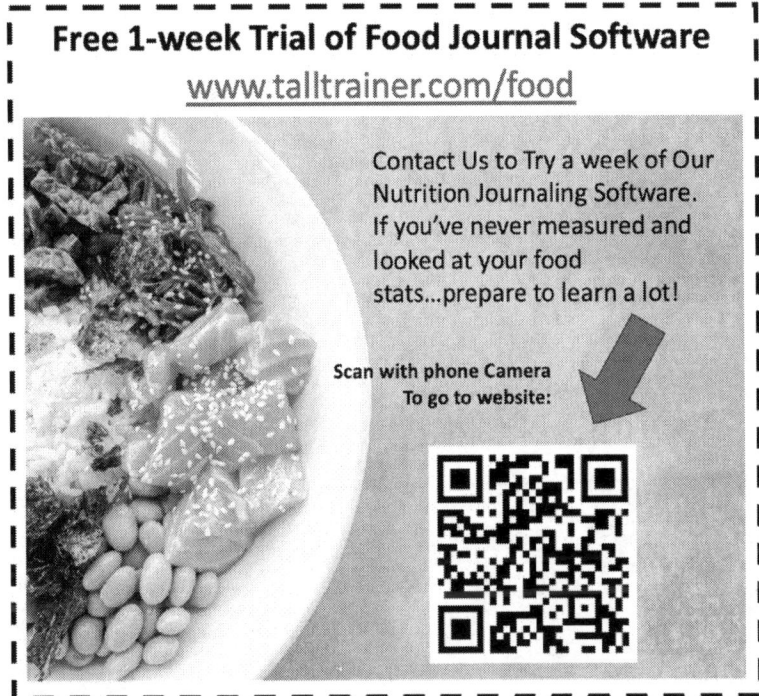

Free 1-week Trial of Food Journal Software
www.talltrainer.com/food

Contact Us to Try a week of Our Nutrition Journaling Software. If you've never measured and looked at your food stats…prepare to learn a lot!

Scan with phone Camera
To go to website:

I have just turned 50 and lost 50 pounds! and I get to eat pizza! (Sally's Results)

Sally can now split squat holding the weight she lost!

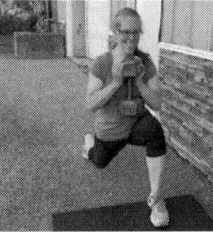

Over 50 POUNDs gone!
-11.5% body fat & <7" @ waist and hips!

WWW.TALLTRAINER.COM

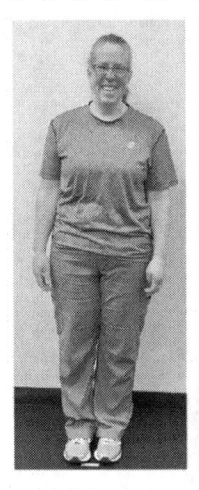
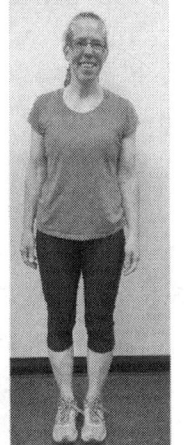
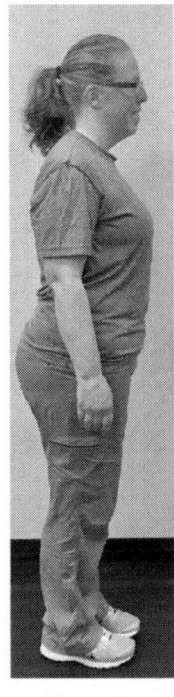
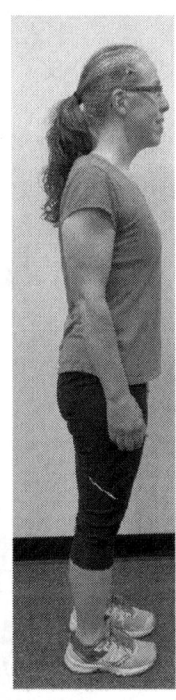

I started my Tall Trainer journey in January of 2020. Prior to starting, I had been mildly active but my nutrition was not great. My weight had been increasing over the years. The only time I had lost weight in the past was if I had kept track of what I ate. Then it would creep back up again. In 2019, I became a grandma- which is THE BEST! I really needed to figure out how to be fit and flexible.

59

I wanted the strength to be able to carry and play with my grandson as he grew. This became my **"WHY?"**

I had heard about Tall Trainer years ago and bought their Fitness in Real Life book- and actually read the whole thing and marked it all up. I looked up the website and decided to call and see if maybe I could join a class.

I was amazed and so thankful for the positive information that I received in that phone call. Stacie (the lady who took my call) was so upbeat and said that they were all **REAL PEOPLE**...who ate pizza! That was a huge selling point as I needed to learn how to manage my cravings with being healthy overall. So I signed up!

The class time was 5:20AM which allowed me to get back home to see my high schoolers off to school. The environment in the class is indescribable. You really have to experience it. Starting class every day with a prayer gets our time together focused. Every day, Gym Class (as I lovingly refer to it) is different. We never know what we will be walking into, which keeps it **super fun**. My class has so many **inspirational people** in it. They are all very kind, supportive and encouraging. *I feel like they are extended family*.

Now, **I have just turned 50 and lost 50 pounds!** It was a great feeling to meet this goal. I have 3 grandchildren and am **more fit then I have ever been in my life.** Plus I have never eaten so well! The VITABOT online food tracker really helps keep me accountable-and I get to eat pizza!

- **Sally**

"If something is too hard for me to do (like the jumping jacks!) or too hard on my mature bones, modifications are made and I'm able to go forward with the workout without losing a step!"

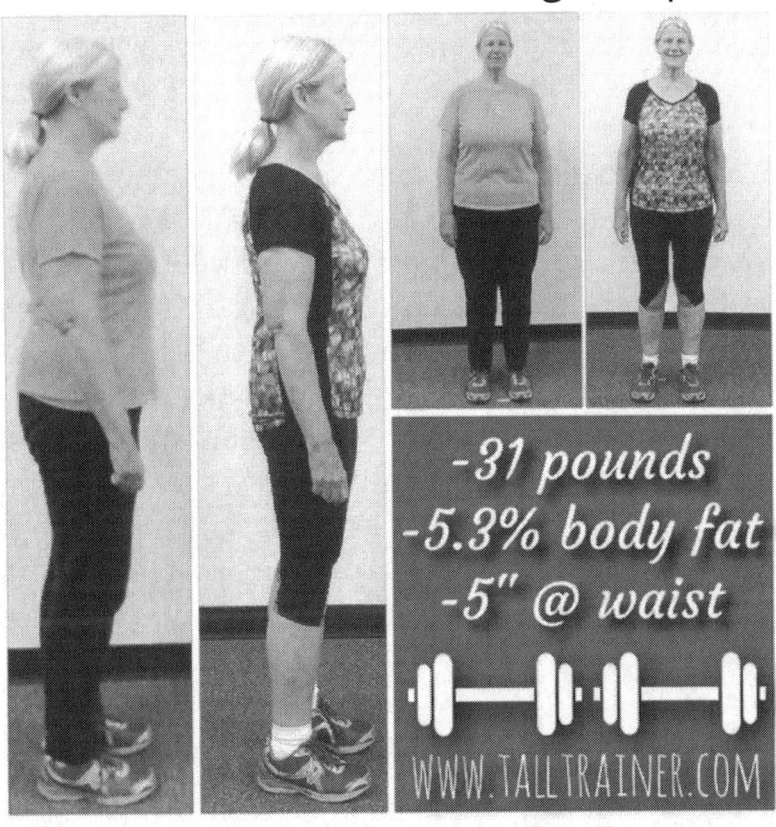

-31 pounds
-5.3% body fat
-5" @ waist

WWW.TALLTRAINER.COM

Prior to last year, I worked in Buffalo for 8 years, staying there during the week. I rented a room from a lady and although I had full access to the kitchen, cooking is not for me. Tried to bring food for the week with me on Monday mornings and it was usually just skimpy salads, sandwiches, cheese & crackers and the like. Easy to make/easy to eat but not too nutritious.

That was my "work life" and when I came home on the weekends I usually stayed home because I was away from home all week. My husband has been doing all the cooking for years now and I've been eating the delicious meals he makes... almost always going back for   seconds!

I started working from home a year ago June and my office just happens to be right around the corner from the refrigerator. By September of last year I started to realize my clothes were getting snug-er and I wasn't doing anything for exercise. I had been seeing the Tall Trainer ads in the Penny Saver for quite a while so I called, took down the information about the program and "filed" it away. Just wasn't ready to take that first step yet. The weather was getting colder and the big, heavy sweaters and oversize winter coats all fit me fine!

Well, come June of this year, I was over 200 lbs, summer was here, I had no clothes that fit me and hadn't exercised in over 2 years. It was time to do something so I called Tall Trainer again. The class time fit into my schedule so I decided to take the leap. And a leap it was!! I remember the first day doing the warm up... jog in place. OK, I can do that. Jumping Jacks... OK I can do that. WAIT A MINUTE!! MY FEET WON'T COME OFF THE GROUND!!! When did I lose the ability to do jumping jacks???? I loved gym class many years

64

ago!! Where did the muscles, flexibility, endurance go all of a sudden?!

Well, after being in boot camp for 6 months now, I'm finding those things again and I love it! I've lost over 30 lbs but that is almost secondary to the strength, confidence and flexibility that I've gained back in such a short time. I realize that you don't lose those things "all of a sudden". It's so true... use it or lose it.

I look forward to boot camp in the mornings and enjoy the camaraderie in the class. Everyone is there for the same purpose - to improve themselves both physically and mentally, with the help of an excellent trainer, Jeremy - and have a lot of fun while doing it! Some days are harder than others but I like that they're all challenging and varied.

If something is too hard for me to do (like the jumping jacks!) or too hard on my mature bones, modifications are made and I'm able to go forward with the workout without losing a step! I have learned so much and have come so far in such a short time, it's amazing.

I would urge anyone of any age to try Tall Trainer for a month. You will definitely notice the difference physically and in attitude at the end of 30 days. If you think you can't, YOU CAN!!

- Kathy

Key #4 – Cardiovascular System Training

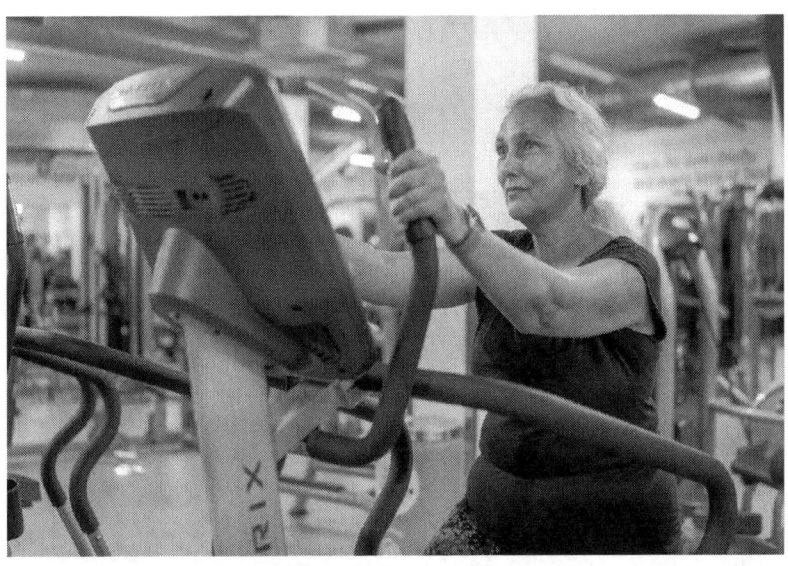

Once you have Resistance Training going well and your nutrition Quality and more importantly Quantity are being watched you can layer in Cardiovascular Training.

Most people do cardio for weight loss. It does help. Every 100 Calories extra you burn per day (without eating more) should get you about a pound of weight loss over a month. 100 Cals x 30 days = 3,000 Calories. There are 3,500 Calories in a Pound.

But you should use nutrition mostly for weight loss. Cardio for a little assistance.

The biggest reason is if you go for a 3 mile walk which takes most people 45 min to 1 hour you'll burn about 300 Calories. If you aren't measuring your food you can take in 300 extra Calories in lunch!

67

So 1 pound of weight loss would be about 35 miles of walking. 5 miles a day 7 days a week. It helps but you still have to watch your nutrition to see that pound truly happen. A lot of people sign up for marathons to get them to run more in an effort to lose weight. There is surprisingly little weight lost unless nutrition is also a focus. You move more you get hungrier and you eat more. Our body likes balancing back out.

I think the main reason for doing cardiovascular exercise should be longevity (living longer) and better energy and vitality.

Longevity and Cardiovascular Exercise

Franklin Booth did a Meta Analysis in 2012 and found that…

"Low cardiorespiratory fitness is a sounder predictor of death then risk factors such as hypertension, smoking, and Diabetes."

A Meta Analysis is when you look at the results of many studies sometimes 20 or 30 or more!

This seems shocking but if you can't walk to the bathroom because of your weak heart and lungs you are just one case of pneumonia away from being gone for good.

CVD, Oxidative stress, Inflammation, & Aging: WHO (2016)

In this World Health Organization research they found Cardiovascular Disease is the #1 cause of death representing 31% of all deaths globally. Surprising since this included starvation in 3rd world countries.

Pioneer Study: Shephard, R. J. (2008). Maximal oxygen intake and independence in old age. British Journal of Sport Medicine Online First, April 10, 2008, pp 1-19

(A Review of 30 studies (since 1990) with male and female subjects age 64 years or older)

What happens as we age?

Men VO2 max tends to drop 5 ml/kg/min each decade after 20 (drop from 45 ml/kg/min)
Women VO2 max tends to drop 5 ml/kg/min each decade after 35 (drop from 38 ml/kg/min)

Decline Largely Due to Inactivity and increase in body fat

Once VO2max drops below 18 (men) 15 (women) a person loses functional independence

Let me clarify these weird numbers. VO2 Max is a measure of how much Oxygen we can use. It's the best measure we have for cardiovascular fitness. It looks like we lose 5 points per decade until it gets so low that someone needs to push us around in a wheel chair.

Now this is what typically happens.

Not what **HAS TO HAPPEN!**

What can we do to stop or reverse this?

Aerobic Activity (50%-70% HRmax; 3-5x a week; 30 min/day) can retard decline. This means basically a walk 3-5 days a week can help us improve this number. For bigger improvements more is needed but most people would get a nice bump doing this.

After…
8-10 weeks – VO2max improves 12.9%
12-18 weeks – VO2max improves 14.1%
24-52 weeks – VO2max improves 16.9%

69

***Higher Intensities (75-85% HRmax) = Greater Gains (25% increase = increase in 6 ml/kg/min)

This is super intense and that makes sense as well because there are people with VO2 Max numbers WAY above the starting average for Men (some twice as high). It can be increased at any time but not without some work!

6 ml/kg/min is *Equivalent to gaining back 12 years of vigor!!!*

I don't use the word vigor often enough but they used it in their results so I think it sounds GREAT!

If you want your VO2 Max to drop just sit in a chair for a month. I bet you can drop a decades worth of points in one month of sitting around!

You'll notice the biggest improvements in this number occurred in the first 8-10 weeks. I think ½ of that or more is gained in the first 4-weeks of adding in this activity.

Also remember that our strength training can get us in the 50-70% HRmax training level so some of our cardio improvements can happen in strength training time. I think we are best served if we get a least 1 really strong and hard interval training workout per week along with our strength training. If you have bunches of time you can add in more cardio workouts but don't take away a strength workout to add in a cardio workout. There's a reason I talked about strength training first!

So, how do I know if I'm in my heart rate zone?

Basically, you feel an increase in breathing. You are starting to breath harder. If you want to play with numbers. The most basic formula for guessing at your max heart rate is 220 – age. So a 50 year old might have a max heart rate around 170. 50% of that is 85 beats per minute. So as long as you are above 85

70

beats (your apple watch might tell you this) or you c
them yourself. Count how many beats in 10 seconds ﹍
it by 6. If you are going for higher intensity 128 beats pᴗ.
minute would put this 50 year old in that 75%+ category.

In our program we add cardio by of course doing resistance
training 2-3x per week. Then 1 high intensity interval day
where we are trying to get above 75% and occasionally 85%
heart rate max so we can maximize improvements. Then we
usually have a lower intensity cardio day that has more
stretching in it that is more in the 65-80% level.

This is a GREAT recipe for long term success and honestly will
probably be my pattern for the rest of my life.

We use different themes and styles for these workouts and
sometimes give them fun names and even a costume or two to
keep it entertaining. Doing the right thing day in and day out
can seem monotonous as times. But, we keep the science of
fitness as a focus while wrapping it in a more fun package.

71

72

Everyone is saying it's impossible to lose weight when you get older

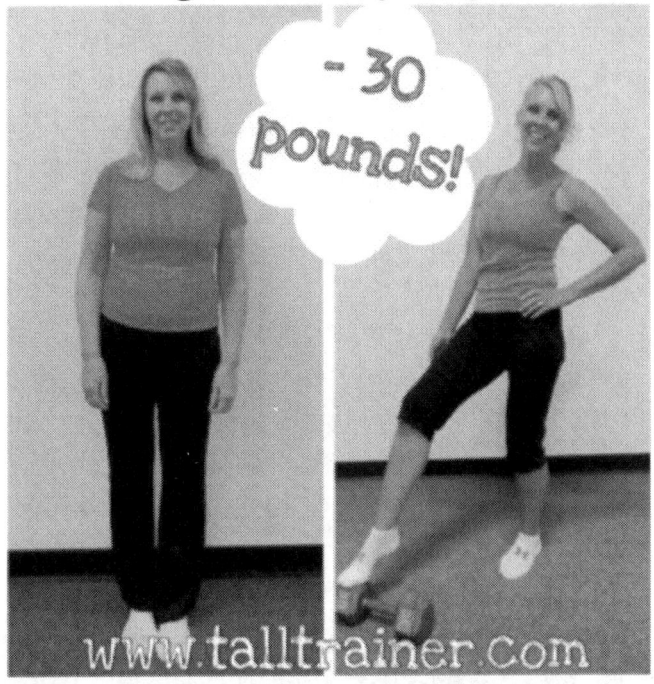

I recently retired from the hospital this past winter. At this new journey I found the opportunity to take time for myself. In the past always working an early start didn't leave me the opportunity to workout before work and often times running to cover for my grandchildren, I didn't take the needed time for myself, what little was left in the day.

I have always been a target for the at home programs, they lure me in, I purchase one and 2 weeks later it's collecting dust. My lack of self-confidence never made me a fan of group exercise. So my comfort level was at home. But I mustered up the courage to try my first

73

'Boot Camp', and the experience has been life changing! ...

As I am right on the heels of turning 60 and everyone saying it's impossible to lose weight when you get older.I knew this was made available to me and all I had to do was show up. I can't put into words the experience I have had, with the program, the people I have met, just the sincere caring of loving people.

There is truly a science of how this all works, but all you have to do is follow the workout Jeremy creates for you. In my first 4 weeks I lost 8 lbs. and 5.5 inches. My second 4 weeks I lost another 7 lbs. and over 5 more inches. To date I am down 30lbs! But my clothes have never fit so nicely.

I'm firmer from head to toe and I have such an inner strength and confidence that has grown from this experience.

My husband says it's his investment in me to continue and he tells me every day how proud he is of me. Four months ago I never would have dreamed this kind of transformation could ever be possible for someone my age. I am living my dream! I deal with a lot of age related ailments but this program helps ease a lot of discomfort you may have and I am pain free. No more slow crawl out of bed.... I jump out, can't wait to get to class. I feel so blessed that I found you, and all your staff. All because I got a postcard in the mail! ♥   - Karen

Real Results
Busy Working Mom Success!

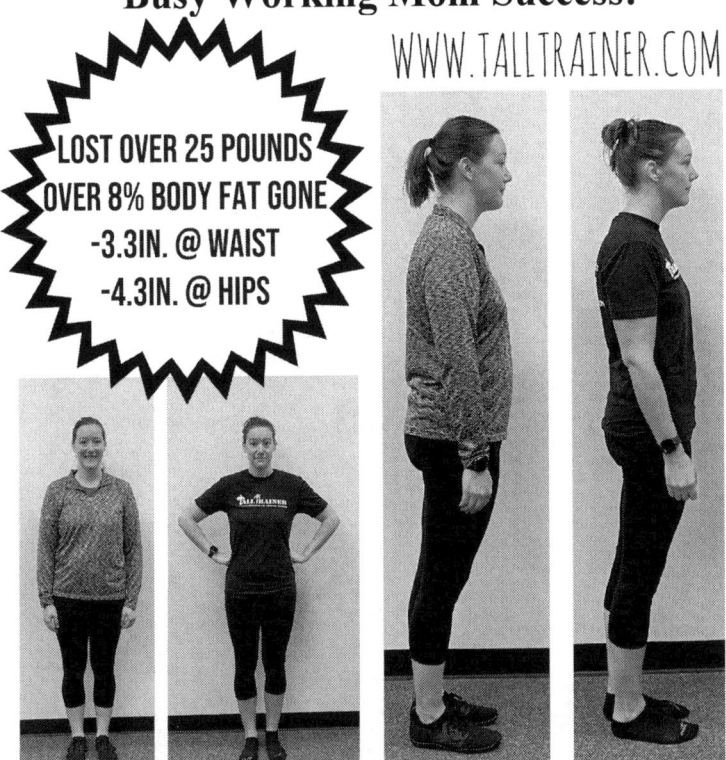

LOST OVER 25 POUNDS
OVER 8% BODY FAT GONE
-3.3IN. @ WAIST
-4.3IN. @ HIPS

I lacked motivation. I was gaining weight, lost my energy, felt tired all the time, and couldn't keep up with my sons. I was constantly anxious and feeling depressed at times. [Cara Joined in June for the summer and has been in class since].

Throughout June, I focused on me, my health and fitness. I fell in love with the routine and became so grateful for the supportive classmates. I was happy to have a time for just myself and have continued in the 5am class since! As of the end of December, **I have lost 30 pounds and over 4 inches off of my core.** I

75

have built my stamina and endurance and found the joy in running again. I'm enjoying and look forward to strength training days and have surprised myself at how much I can push myself and the amount that I can lift.

I have more daily energy and am enjoying finding more outdoor/physical activities to do with my sons. **By putting my nutrition and fitness as a priority, I have also seen a shift with my husband and sons.** They want to be physically active with me more, drink more water and have begun to learn more about their nutrition too.

- Cara

#5 – Mobility or Flexibility Training

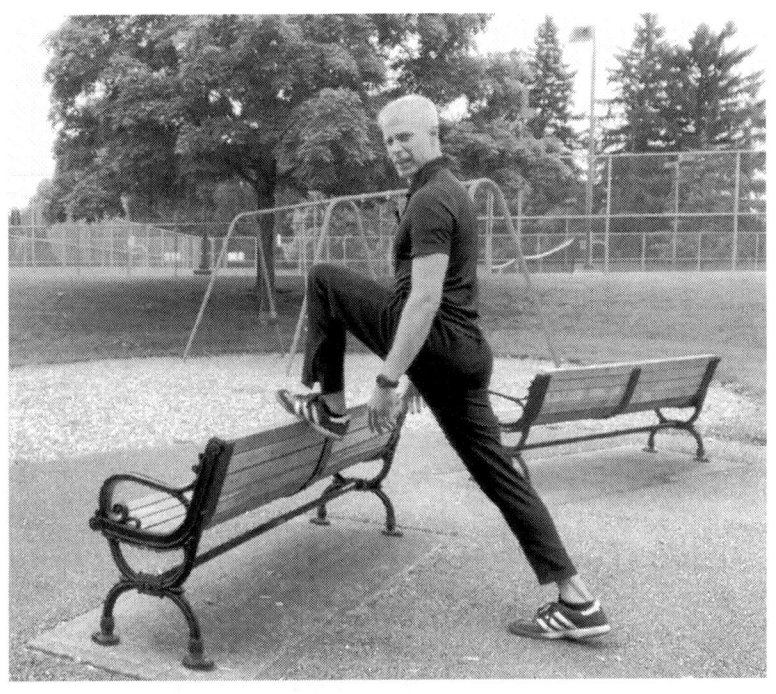

You won't regret time spent in this area. This area is often an after thought. Most people skip their stretching time consistently. Now mobility is more than stretching and I'll cover some of this.

First, I need to explain how this became important to me…

I was 22 years old and a college pole vaulter. I ruptured a disc in my lower back. Basically, just popped it out like a grape. I spent 6-months doing bunch of nothing on doctors orders. It just kept hurting, only after 6-months I was weak and depressed too. I felt MUCH older than 22. In this process I realized…

77

"The more flexible you are the younger you feel"

I was SOOO TIGHT. Mostly hamstring but all around my hips as well. I was training hard but not well balanced and I didn't want to "over stretch" so I never stretched very far or long for that matter.

It caught up to me and took me several years of learning to find my way out of it. Now you wouldn't be able to tell I have a back issue. My flexibility (and strength) keeps it away.

Here's my best sales pitch for stretching.

Imagine whenever you sit down a giant spider starts spinning webs around your body. The longer you sit there the thicker the webs get. If you don't get up and **MOVE** and **USE** your **FULL RANGE OF MOTION** you will lose the ability to. The webs will be too tight to break. This is not far from the truth. Our body is always rebuilding and will take the shape we put it in most often. Most of us don't want to turn out like a slouch but it happens more often than not.

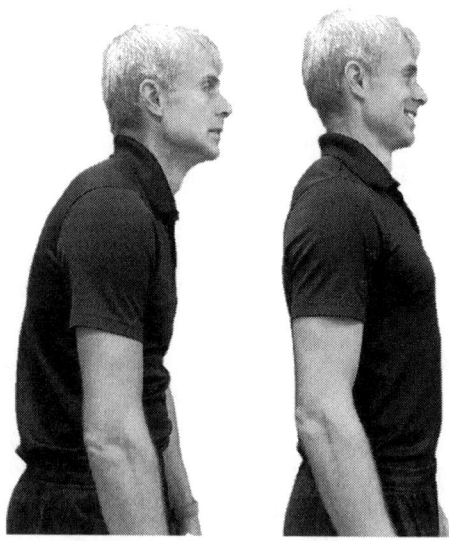

78

It's this factor that causes the most joint pain and problems. I think a full 50% of joint issues can be solved by stretching. That's a lot of what happens in physical therapy! When an area gets tight it puts pressure on other areas.

Stability and Mobility Zones

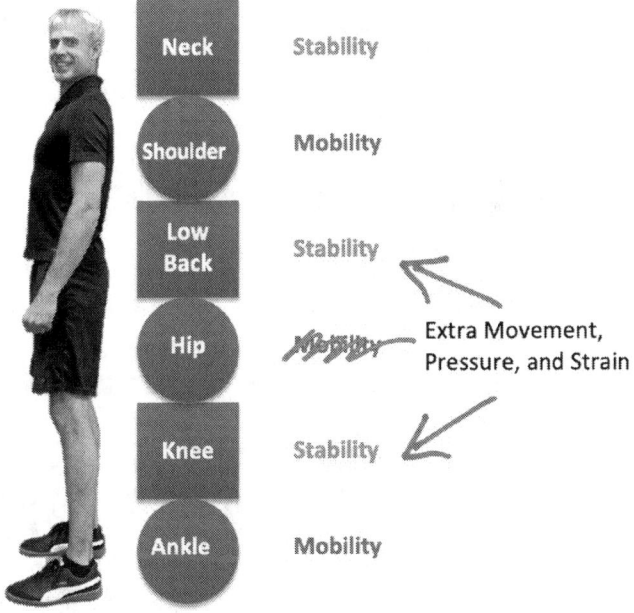

The 3 areas that tighten the most are:
- Shoulders
- Hips
- Ankles (calves)

When the shoulders tighten too much they put pressure on the neck, rotator cuff, and lower back. When the hips tighten too much they put pressure on knees, back, and feet. When the ankles tighten too much they put pressure on feet (plantar fasciitis), knees, and some back too.

If we can strengthen and stretch these 3 areas it could get us feeling decades younger and make everyday life a whole lot easier.

How to get flexible and "younger"

1.) **Exercise with great posture and as much range of motion as you can while maintaining posture.** Our best stretches are often our strength training exercises. The reason for this is standard stretching only adds a minimal amount of flexibility. The body often won't let you stretch farther if you don't have the strength to protect yourself. You don't want your arm falling off!

2.) **Stretch Daily or at least after each workout.** Break the webbing daily to keep it from getting too tight or at least to stop it from getting tighter. Often our weakness is caused by fighting our own tightness while trying to move or lift.

3.) **Have a day each week with more stretching.** Our muscles do well with longer stretch time. Just like resistance training takes multiple sets so does stretching. Getting more like 2 minutes total per muscle will have a better effect than 30 seconds or less. You can do it in sets of 30 seconds still but repeating 3-4x to accumulate the 2 minutes worth.

4.) **If you already have an injury or pain stretch/exercise more.** If your webbing is already locked in tight it's going to take some extra work. More stretching and exercising and perhaps massage to get the tense tissues to soften, stretch, and become more elastic.

Here are some pictures of some basic stretches that would be wise to add into your routine. These or something like them!

(see next page)

BASIC STRETCHING REFERENCE SHEET

Hold each stretch for 30 seconds each side.

Lying Down

| 1.) Knee In Stretch | 2.) Hip/Butt Stretch |

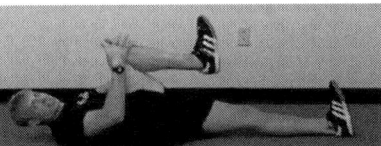 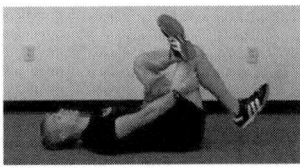

Standing

| 3.) Triceps Stretch | 4.) Hamstring | 5.) Front Hip |

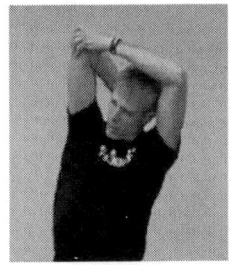 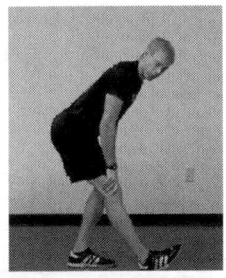 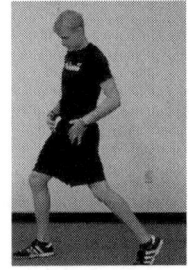

Standing By Wall

| 6.) Quad | 7.) Calf Stretch | 8.) Chest Stretch |

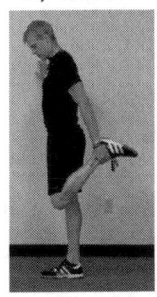 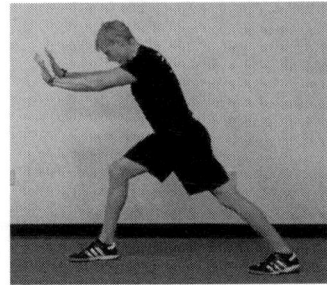 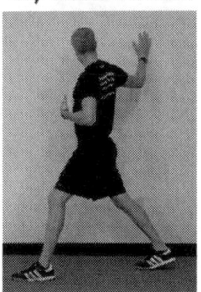

How do we use this in our program?

In our program we stretch at the end of every class. A bit longer than a typical fitness class. We have one day a week with a little more stretching. And we certainly work on doing our exercises in a way that creates the biggest benefit. Sometimes subtle adjustments can make big differences. In 1-on-1 training we finish every workout with an assisted stretch because you can make progress faster when you have help stretching.

For more stretching resources please contact us with some of your specific challenges, there might even be a video we have made that we can send you to help!

Summary

So that's all I plan to say right now. Here's the recap.

If you want to feel better you need to…

- Do Resistance Training
- Do Some More Resistance Training
- Understand the power of Quantity of Food (and quality a little too)
- Train your Cardiovascular System
- Bend, Move, and Stretch

I wrote this book to be a helpful guide.

Some people will read this and instantly start doing these things.

That's not me…

I have the best intentions and desire but life sometimes distracts me too. I don't LOVE EXERCISE or BROCCOLI. I have to set up habits and put myself in a program with accountability to someone else so I follow through on my best intentions.

This is why I become a personal trainer.

I saw that people like me need a program to keep their commitments to themselves. They need exercise to be more fun. And they need reminders and encouragement to improve their eating habits.

If you are a go and do consistently without fail you should probably go and do that. You'd still love our classes but it wouldn't be as life transforming for you.

But,

83

If you struggle to stay on a program. Not sure where to start. Plan to exercise more than you do. Or find yourself eating more than you know you should. Maybe we can team up with you and help.

We have a 100% money back guarantee that says you'll be amazed at the results you get in your first month.

If you are interested please call us: 585-260-4235
Or fill out a form on our website: www.talltrainer.com

You can even email me directly @ jeremy@talltrainer.com

It is our passion to help people like you feel better!

Lost over 40 pounds, at least 7 inches each from my chest, waist and hips, nearly 12% body fat and have never felt better!

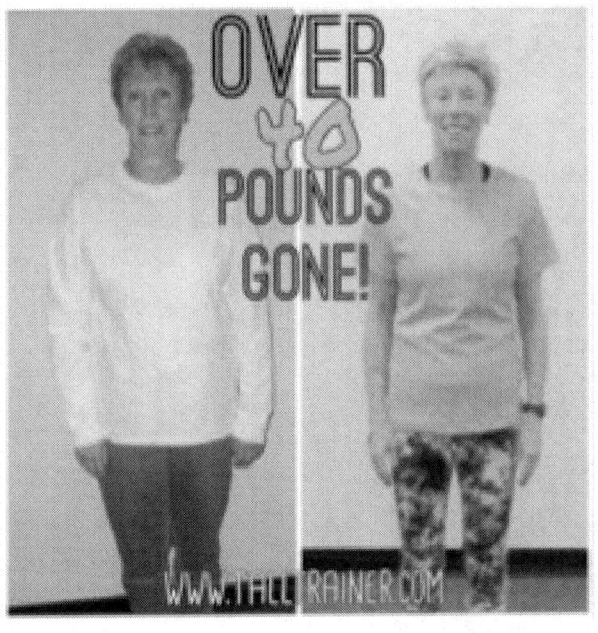

The journey that led me to Tall Trainer began 3 years ago. I had gone through some serious medical issues; we sold our house, moved to the Finger Lakes and built our retirement home all in the span of 1 1/2 years. However, by this time I was exhausted physically and mentally, and knew I needed to make another change in my life....this time, one that would put me in a position where I could enjoy what opportunities life now held for me.

In the fall of 2013, I saw a cover ad on the local Penny Saver telling about a fitness program called "Tall Trainer".....it sounded interesting, but at the time I wasn't quite ready to make a commitment to add another element to my life that would require more time and effort. So the cover page sat on my tabletop for a few more months as the pounds accumulated and the energy level sank...

In January of 2014 I was ready to take control of my life once again. After all, I thought, this is the only life I'll get so I might as well start making it the best one I could! And so I called the number from the Penny Saver ad. I signed up for a month to see if this was what would help me get back on track to the life I wanted and needed.

The first month was full of ups and downs, struggles and victories. It wasn't easy for a 62 year old, who had been fairly active for most of her life, to realize that jumping jacks, slide-backs, push-ups and squats were NOT things that improved with age! But at the end of the month, after gaining friends and some self-confidence, losing over 5 pounds and 3% body fat, I thought that I'd try it for another month.....and then another, and then another. I've now been with Tall Trainer for over 1 1/2 years, and have lost over 40 pounds, at least 7 inches each from my chest, waist and hips, nearly 12% body fat and have never felt better!

My eating habits are greatly improved through the education that Jeremy provides as well as the Vitabot program utilized by Tall Trainer to which every member has access. It was such a strong factor in helping me attain my goal weight. It helps individuals create meal plans to meet their objectives and goals, and educates users as to nutritional values of various foods. Long live veggies!

I am convinced that this is where I was meant to be, that a powerful force in my life guided me to this program and these exceptional people who have strengthened me physically, mentally and spiritually. The motivation and encouragement given by Jeremy and his staff gives me an inner drive to work hard, and to succeed.

They educate their boot camp members so that safety is always a factor as exercises are performed. Variety in our daily regimen really provides incentive to attend each day. Boxing is one of my favorite "stations", as I'd never done that before! What a stress reliever!! And weights are another favorite....what an immediate awareness of self-improvement as you increase the amount you can lift! I'm also doing my push-ups from my toes....not many, but OK for a 64 year old!!

Also, I treasure the way Jeremy works to keep our sessions interesting for boot campers; seeing the staff in President's Day costumes, our spooky Halloween work-outs with a pumpkin, and Jeremy in a grass skirt, just for the fun of it!!! What a talented, knowledgeable and dedicated group of men and women, we are so fortunate to have them guiding us, teaching us, and caring about us. They are so uniquely great!

I am so thankful to be a part of Tall Trainer. The friendships that have developed will last because we all share similar journeys through life. I've gone on far too long, and want to wrap this up by saying "thank you" to Tall Trainer. Your value is immeasurable, and the lives you've changed so very many. We're so blessed you're in our lives!   - Deb

(It's been 10 years and Deb is still an amazing role model! Just saw her today kicking butt!)

Ok, so you read this far...

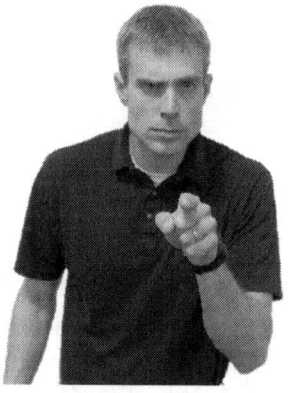

I really want to work with motivated people like you. We know we can't be the most help unless someone is ready to take action themselves.

By reading this book you have taken a BIG step. And we at Tall Trainer Fitness would love to help you.

So, if you go to our website and fill out the form. Type the phrase, "Time to Shine".

And we'd like to give you a discount on your first month with us.

**Scan with phone Camera
To go to website:**

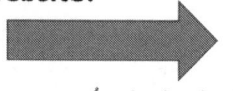

www.talltrainer.com/get-started

www.talltrainer.com

Thank you for Reading!

May God bless you and your health now and forever!

www.talltrainer.com